THRIVE ENERGY COOKBOOK

150 FUNCTIONAL, PLANT-BASED WHOLE FOOD RECIPES

BRENDAN BRAZIER

PENGUIN
an imprint of Penguin Canada Books Inc., a Penguin Random House Company

Published by the Penguin Group
Penguin Canada Books Inc., 90 Eglinton Avenue East, Suite 700, Toronto, Ontario, Canada
M4P 2Y3

Penguin Group (USA) Inc., 375 Hudson Street, New York, New York 10014, U.S.A.
Penguin Books Ltd, 80 Strand, London WC2R 0RL, England
Penguin Ireland, 25 St Stephen's Green, Dublin 2, Ireland (a division of Penguin Books Ltd)
Penguin Group (Australia), 707 Collins Street, Melbourne, Victoria 3008, Australia (a division of
Pearson Australia Group Pty Ltd)
Penguin Books India Pvt Ltd, 11 Community Centre, Panchsheel Park, New Delhi – 110 017, India
Penguin Group (NZ), 67 Apollo Drive, Rosedale, Auckland 0632, New Zealand (a division of
Pearson New Zealand Ltd)
Penguin Books (South Africa) (Pty) Ltd, 24 Sturdee Avenue, Rosebank, Johannesburg 2196,
South Africa

Penguin Books Ltd, Registered Offices: 80 Strand, London WC2R 0RL, England

First published 2014

1 2 3 4 5 6 7 8 9 10 (CR)

Photography: Kevin Clark
Food & Prop Styling: Jennifer Stamper
Production Assistant: Monique Cheung

Special thanks for photography pre-production assistance:
Robin del Pino, Byron Gronseth, Christine Berube, Phyllis Chu, Meera Bennett

Additional photography on pages xiv-xv by Dan Barham; pages 104-105,
125, and 148-149 by Brendan Brazier; inside front and back covers and
pages 28-29, 254-255, and 258-259 by Rob Campbell; pages 201 and 278 by
Stephanie D'Cunha; pages 16-17 and 280 by Donovan Jenkins; page xxvi by
Jonnie Karan; pages 274-275 by Melissa Schwartz

Manufactured in the U.S.A.

Library and Archives Canada Cataloguing in Publication

Brazier, Brendan, author
Thrive energy cookbook / Brendan Brazier.

Includes index.
ISBN 978-0-14-318707-3 (pbk.)

1. Vegan cooking. 2. Cooking (Natural foods). 3. Food allergy–
Diet therapy–Recipes. 4. Cookbooks. I. Title.

TX837.B724 2014   641.5'636   C2013-905145-7

Visit the Penguin Canada website at **www.penguin.ca**

Special and corporate bulk purchase rates available; please see **www.penguin.ca/corporatesales**
or call 1-800-810-3104, ext. 2477.

To my Grandma, Helen Brazier, who led by example.
Seen here in 1942, cycling over Lions Gate Bridge in Vancouver.

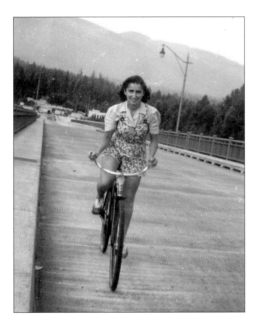

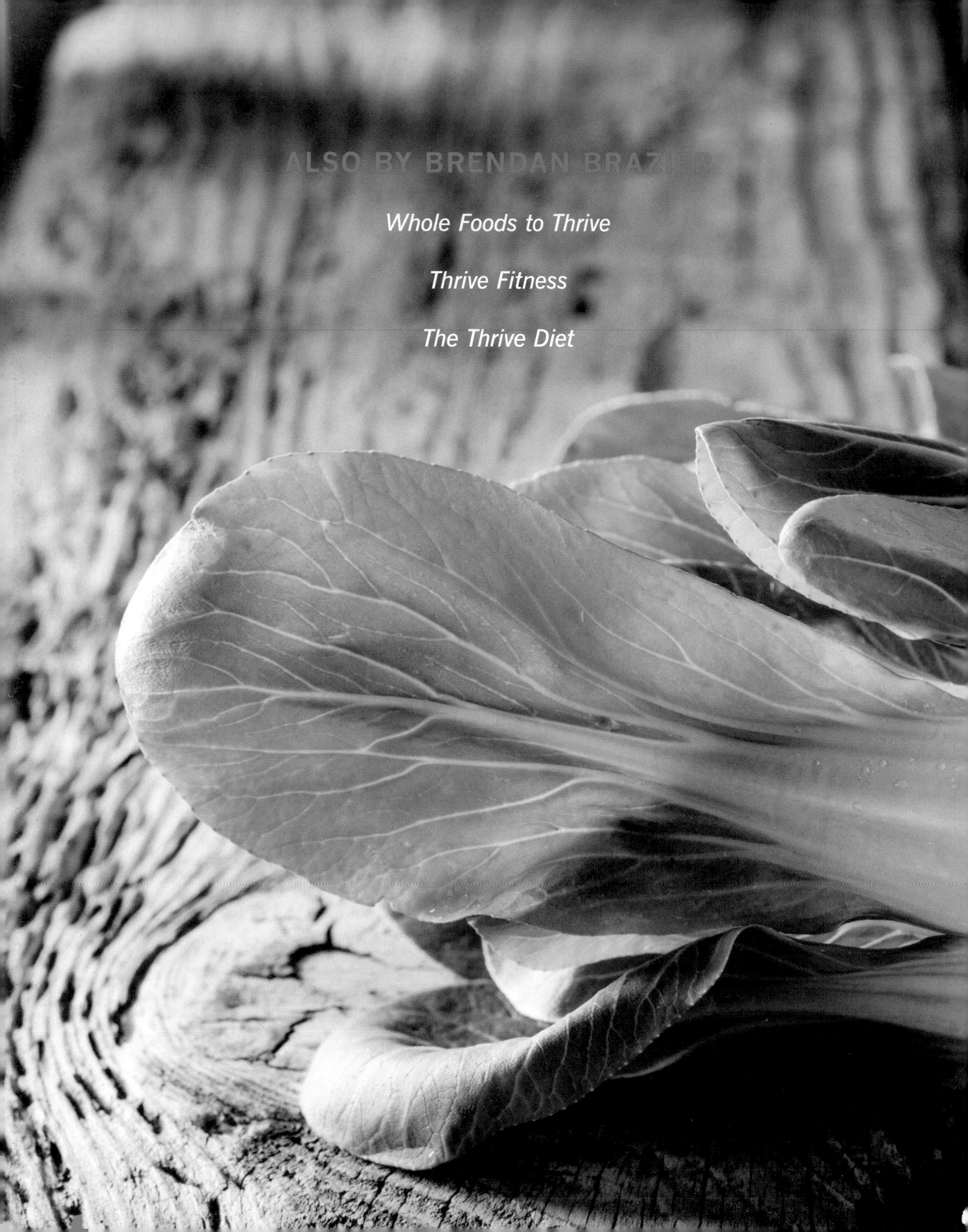

ALSO BY BRENDAN BRAZIER

Whole Foods to Thrive

Thrive Fitness

The Thrive Diet

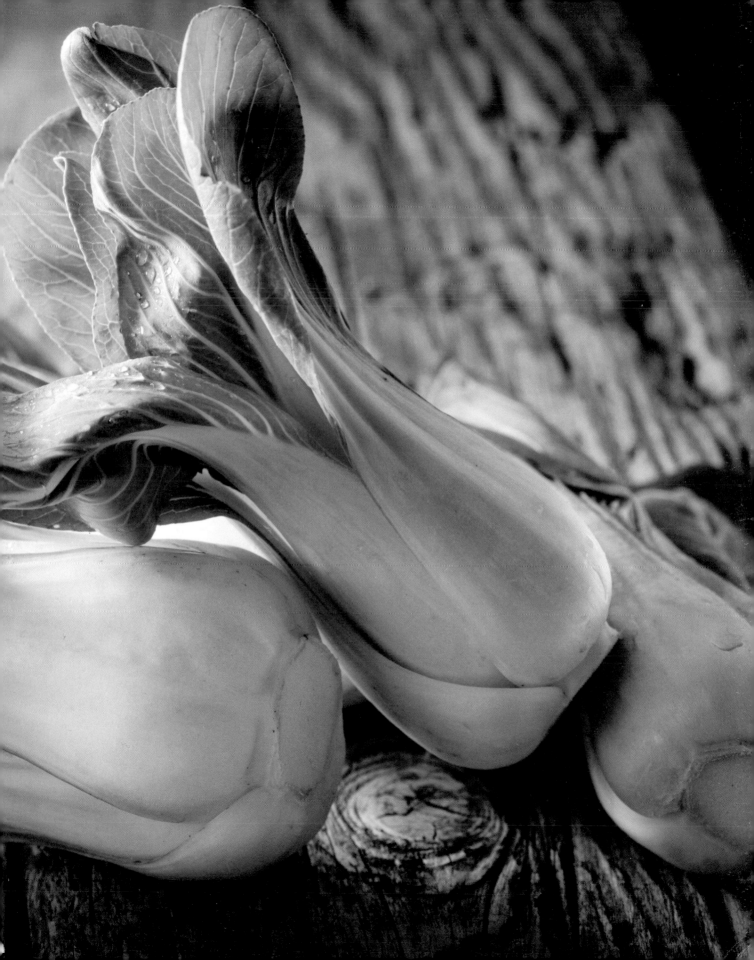

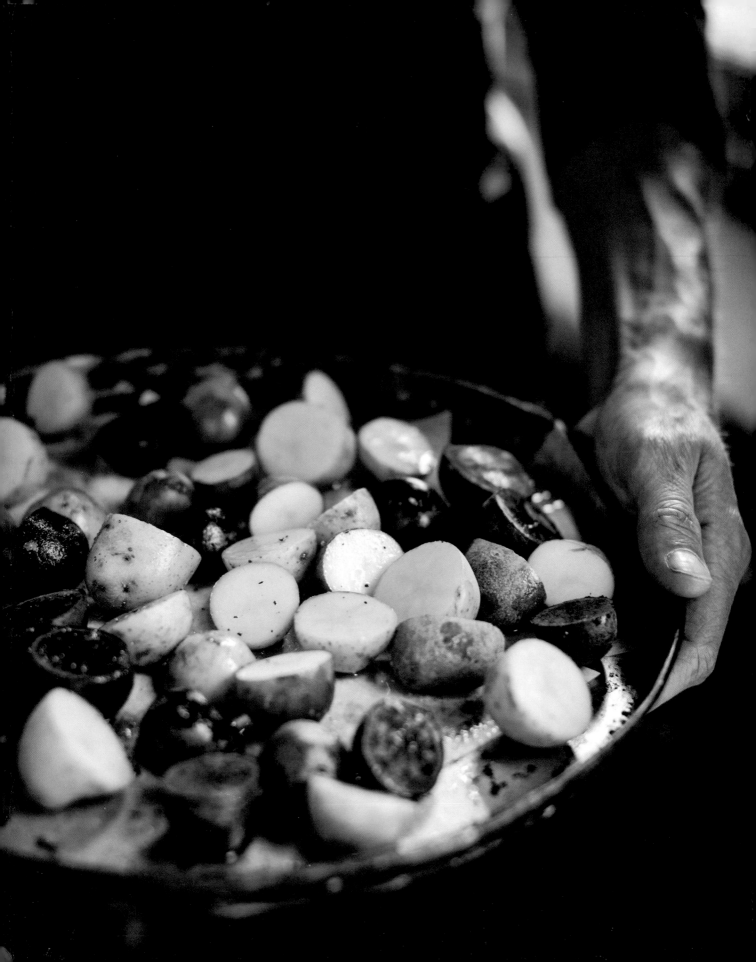

CONTENTS

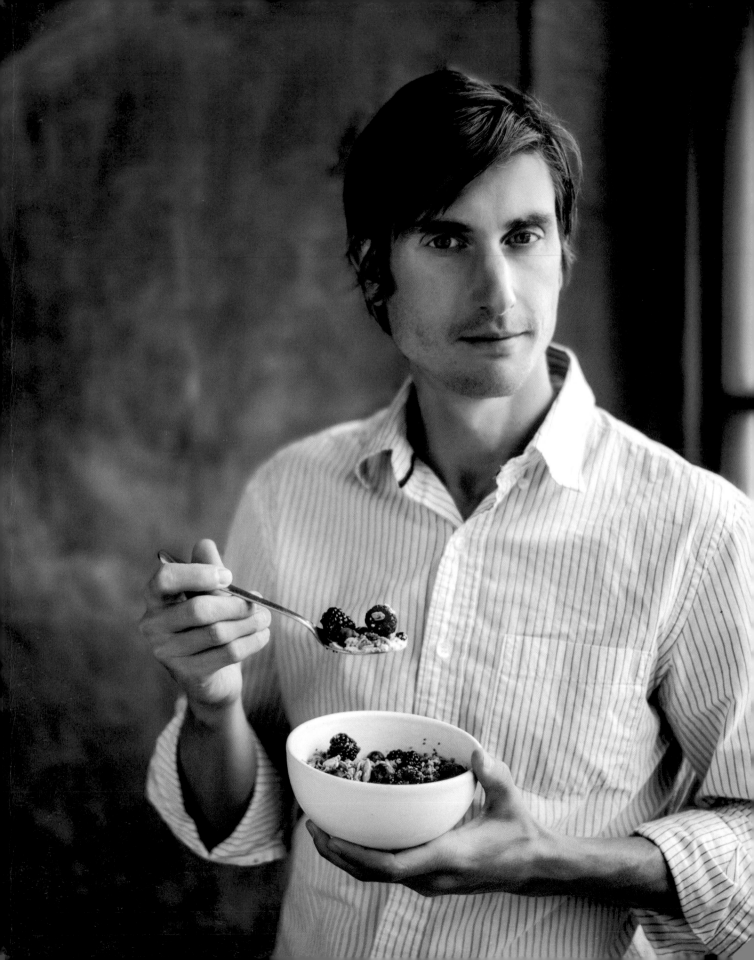

My Thrive Journey: Purpose-driven, clean, plant-based nutrition

What follows is a brief overview of my approach to clean, plant-based nutrition that I introduced in my first book, *The Thrive Diet.* I intend it to serve as a quick refresher if you are already eating the Thrive way. However, if you are eating a traditional North American diet and aim to revamp it, or even just fine-tune your already solid nutrition plan, this section can serve as your introduction to my Thrive philosophy: plant-based, whole food, high-net-gain, and alkaline-forming, without creating biological debt. If you'd like to delve deeper into these topics, you may want to consider reading *The Thrive Diet.* It expands on these subjects in great detail.

When I was fifteen and beginning to train for triathlon, it took hundreds of thousands of swim strokes, pedal rotations, and running strides before I could even begin to race Ironman. I didn't put in much mental effort. I simply went out and swam, cycled, and ran. It was a basic, haphazard approach, but it worked—I got better. Yet I noticed that as I continued to improve over the years, my rate of improvement slowed. It became clear to me that my workouts needed to be better targeted to what I was trying to achieve. They had to have purpose.

So I developed a systematic training program. I approached my workouts with purpose and intent for each session. I had a specific goal for every workout, with regard to both what I intended to put into it and what I wanted to get in return. And it worked. My routines yielded quicker gains. I continued to improve, but this time, the rate at which the gains came stayed steady. This was a breakthrough for me. I realized that purpose and intent in all energy expended return a greater level of fitness than I could ever have imagined.

I began looking at other aspects of my program with the same critical eye. Was there purpose and intent in all aspects of my training? I saw clearly that there wasn't. And, as I now shrewdly realized, that lack directly translated into a loss of potential. With this purpose-and-intent mindset now firmly ingrained, I began evaluating what I ate. I considered how my diet affected my training and whether it was mindful eating. When I ate something, what did I hope to get in return? Was it more energy? Was it inflammation reduction? Was it greater rate of recovery? Was it going to affect my ability to get a deep, restorative sleep? Was it going to help me build lean, functional muscle? If I didn't know why I was eating—other than because I was hungry—I asked myself, what gain is this going to give me, and is that what I need right now? Could I make a better choice that would further my progress more quickly?

For example, some foods are best eaten as fuel, before a workout, while others are ideally consumed immediately after a workout to help along the recovery process and rebuild what the exercise broke down. In the competitive sport world, knowing the difference and eating accordingly can mean the difference between success and failure. For that reason, in this book I include a sport-specific section with recipes I formulated specifically to help you prepare for, sustain, and recover from a workout.

Eating with purpose and mindfulness became an integral part of my training and therefore of my daily life. And, as with purposeful training, intentioned eating advanced my rate of improvement in leaps and bounds. And it wasn't just training that this purpose-driven nutrition benefited. Every aspect of life became easier. The quality of my sleep improved, my mental clarity increased, my ability to handle stress and not get sick kicked in. This was far-reaching holistic progress.

Thrive Energy recipes are built with intent, and therefore function is the result. They are purpose driven to give you the nutritional building blocks you need to fuel performance—mental and physical—and reap the rewards of mindful eating. The positive impact for me has been immense.

Like me, many people when they are starting out don't know what foods to eat, how to combine them synergistically, or when to eat them. But it's not complicated. Eat a plant-based whole foods diet—that's essentially it. With a few small tweaks, that diet can bolster results above and beyond.

To help me make informed food choices, I keep in mind three overarching nutritional objectives. These form the core of the Thrive Energy philosophy.

- High-net-gain nutrition
- Alkaline-forming foods
- Elimination of biological debt

Go for High-Net-Gain Foods: Make a small investment for a big return

High-net-gain foods, such as leafy greens and colorful vegetables, deliver energy by way of conservation rather than consumption. Here's what I mean by that. The digestive and assimilation process is an energy-intensive one. As soon as we start eating, we begin spending digestive energy to convert the energy stored within food—also known as calories—into usable sustenance to meet our biological requirements. Whenever energy is transferred from one form to another, there's some loss of energy. However, the amount of energy lost in this process varies greatly depending on the foods eaten.

Highly processed, refined, denatured food requires that significantly more digestive energy be spent to break it down in the process of transferring its caloric energy to us:

net energy gain = energy remaining once digestive energy has been spent

While it's true that a calorie is a measure of food energy, simply eating more calories does not necessarily ensure more energy for the consumer. If there were such a calorie guarantee, people who subsisted on fast food and other such calorie-laden fare would have abundant energy. And of course they don't. And that just points to the excessive amount of digestive energy required to convert such food into usable fuel. (Digestion is tiring. It's no coincidence that the cultures that have their largest, heaviest meals at lunch are the same ones that have afternoon siestas.)

"The less energy spent on digestion, the more energy you'll have."

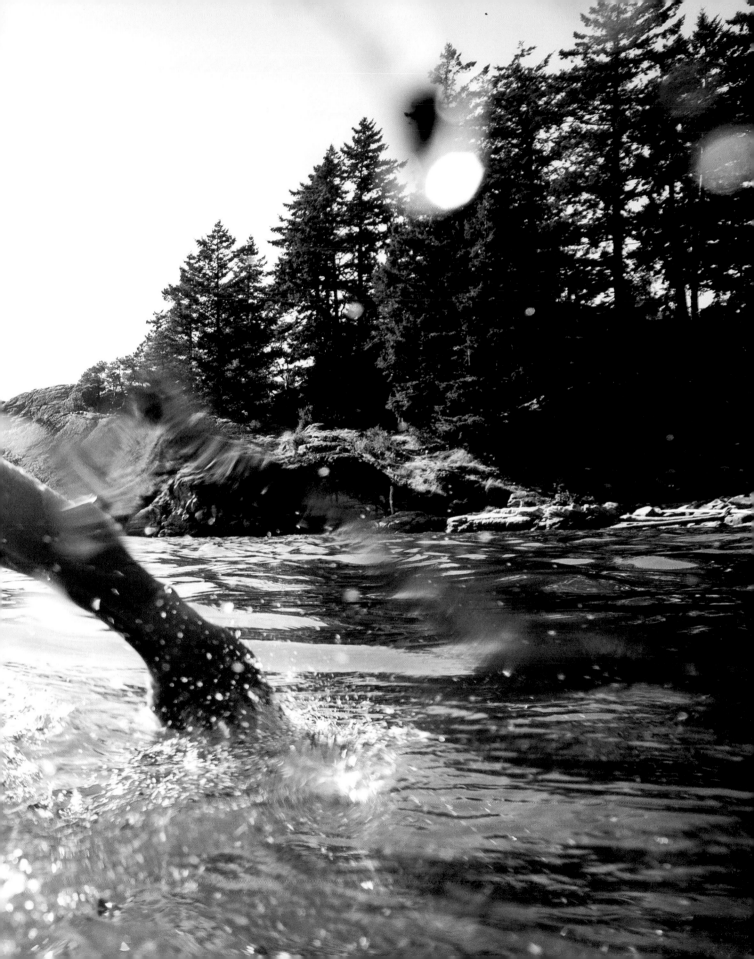

In contrast, natural, unrefined whole food requires considerably less energy to digest. Therefore, we gain more usable energy when we eat foods that are in a more natural whole state, even if they have fewer calories.

Once I grasped this concept, I began viewing my food consumption as though it were an investment. My goal became to spend, or invest, as little digestive energy as possible to acquire the greatest amount of micronutrients and maximize the return on my investment. For this reason, I refer to foods that require little digestive energy but yield a healthy dose of micronutrients as high-net-gain foods:

high net gain = little digestive energy spent, substantial level of micronutrients gained

With this principle in mind, I suggest shifting carbohydrate sources from processed and refined carbs such as pasta and bread to fruits and pseudograins instead. Fruits and pseudograins are packed with carbohydrates in the form of easily assimilated carbs, and they are considerably easier to digest than refined grain flour. As well, both provide a higher micronutrient level than processed, refined carb sources.

Choose Alkaline-Forming Foods

The measure of acidity or alkalinity is called pH, and maintaining a balanced pH within the body is an important part of achieving and sustaining peak health. If our pH drops, our body becomes too acidic, adversely affecting health at the cellular level. People with low pH are prone to many ailments and to fatigue.

The body can become more acidic because of diet and, to a lesser extent, stress. Since our body has buffering capabilities, our blood pH will generally vary only a small degree, regardless of poor diet or other types of stress. But the other systems recruited to aid with this buffering use energy and can become strained. Over time, the result of this buffering is significant stress on the system, which causes immune function to falter, effectively opening the door to a host of illnesses.

Low body pH can lead to the development of kidney stones, the loss of bone mass, and a reduction of growth hormone. And since a decline in growth hormone directly results in loss of lean muscle tissue and increased body fat, the overconsumption of acid-forming foods plays a significant role in North America's largest health crisis. However, food is not the only thing we put in our bodies that is acid-forming. Most prescription drugs, artificial sweeteners, and synthetic vitamin and mineral supplements are extremely acid-forming.

Low body pH is also responsible for an increase in the fabrication of cell-damaging free radicals and a loss in cellular energy production. Free radicals alter cell membranes and can adversely affect our DNA.

So what can we do to prevent all this? The answer is to consume more alkaline-forming foods and fewer acid-forming ones. Minerals are exceptionally alkaline-forming, so foods with a greater concentration of micronutrients—those with greater nutrient density—will inherently have a greater alkaline-forming effect.

Another factor that significantly raises the pH of food and, in turn, the body is chlorophyll content. Responsible for giving plants their green pigment, chlorophyll is often referred to as the blood of plants. The botanical equivalent of hemoglobin in human blood, chlorophyll synthesizes energy. Chlorophyll converts the sun's energy that is absorbed by the plant into carbohydrate. This process, known as photosynthesis, is responsible for life on Earth. Since animals and humans eat plants, we too get our energy from the sun, plants being the conduit. Chlorophyll is prized for its ability to cleanse our blood by helping remove toxins deposited from dietary and environmental sources. Chlorophyll is also linked to the body's production of red blood cells, making daily consumption of chlorophyll-rich foods important for ensuring our body's constant cell regeneration and for improving oxygen transport in the body and, therefore, energy levels. By optimizing the body's regeneration of blood cells, chlorophyll also contributes to peak athletic performance.

pH Effect of Selected Thrive Diet Foods

Foods	Highly Alkaline-Forming	Alkaline-Forming	Neutral	Slightly Acid-Forming
Vegetables	• Asparagus • Beets • Bell peppers • Broccoli • Carrots • Cauliflower • Celery • Chicory • Cucumbers • Dill • Dulse • Green beans • Leafy greens • Leeks • Onion • Parsley • Parsnips • Peas • Sea vegetables • Sprouts (all) • Zucchini	• Squash • Sweet potatoes • Yams		
Pseudograins		• Amaranth • Buckwheat • Millet • Quinoa • Wild rice		
Legumes				• Adzuki beans • Black beans • Black-eyed peas • Chickpeas • Lentils
Seeds		• Sesame	• Flax • Hemp • White chia	• Pumpkin • Sunflower

pH Effect of Selected Thrive Diet Foods

Foods	Highly Alkaline-Forming	Alkaline-Forming	Neutral	Slightly Acid-Forming
Fruit	• Grapefruit • Lemons • Limes • Mangoes • Melons (most) • Papayas	• Apples • Avocados • Bananas • Berries (most) • Cantaloupe • Cherries • Dates • Figs • Grapes • Nectarines • Oranges • Peaches • Pears • Persimmons • Pineapple • Pomegranates		
Oils		• Flaxseed • Hemp • Pumpkin seed	• Coconut	
Nuts		• Almonds • Coconut	• Macadamia • Walnuts	
Grains				• Brown rice • Oats • Spelt
Flours			• Amaranth • Buckwheat • Quinoa	
Sweeteners	• Stevia		• Agave nectar • Coconut nectar	
Miscellaneous	• Gingerroot • Green tea • Herbs, fresh (general) • Rooibos • Yerba mate	• Balsamic vinegar • Cider vinegar • Garlic	• Herbs, dried (general) • Miso paste • Spices (general)	

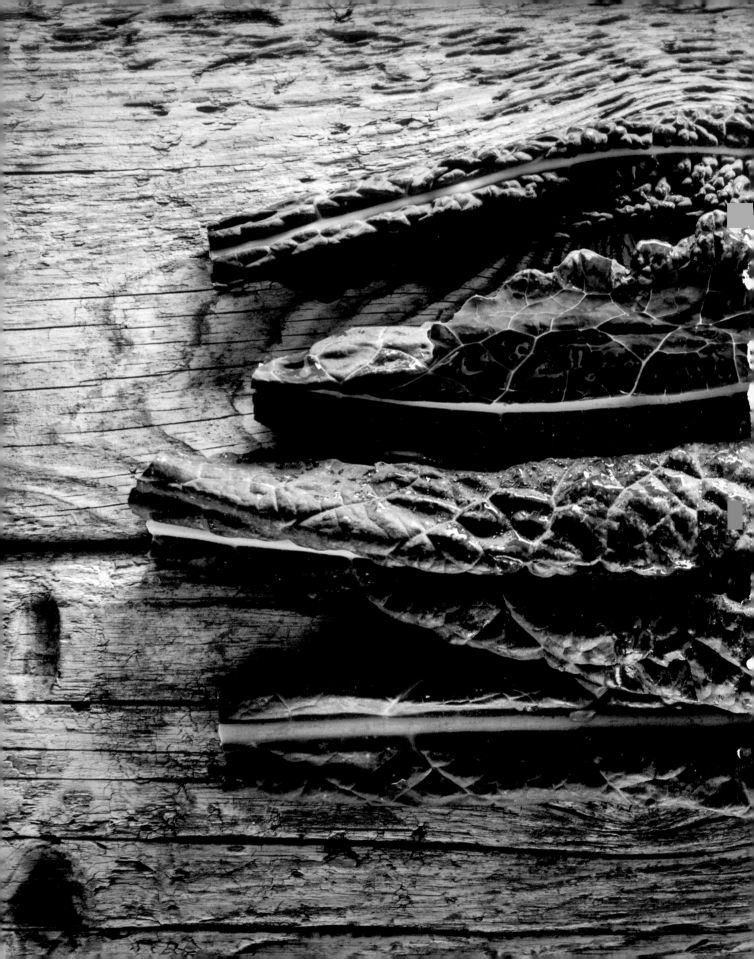

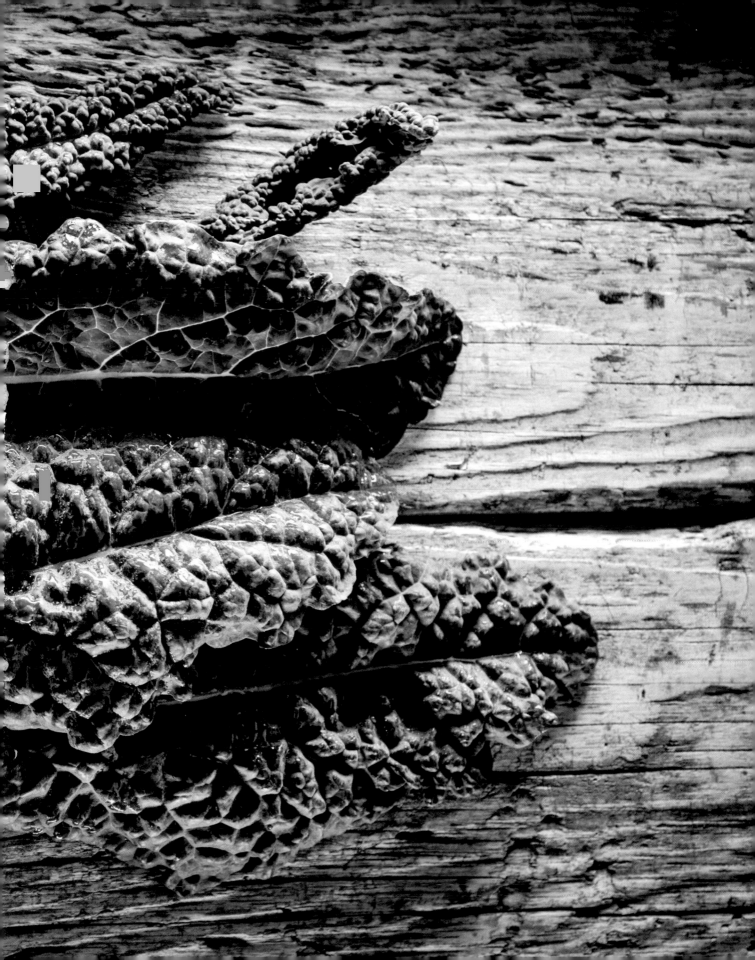

Eliminate Biological Debt: Acquire energy through nourishment, not stimulation

"Biological debt" is the term I use to describe the unfortunate energy-depleted state that North Americans frequently find themselves in. Often brought about by eating refined sugar or drinking coffee to gain short-term energy, biological debt is the ensuing energy crash.

There are two types of energy: one obtained from stimulation, the other obtained from nourishment. The difference between the two is clear cut. Stimulation is short-term energy and simply treats the symptom of fatigue. Being well nourished, in contrast, eliminates the need for stimulation, because a steady supply of energy is available to those whose nutritional needs have been met. In effect, sound nutrition is a pre-emptive strike against fatigue and the ensuing desire for stimulants. With nutrient-dense whole food as the foundation of your diet, there's no need to ever get into biological debt.

Generally speaking, the more a food is fractionalized (the term used to describe a once-whole food that has had nutritional components removed), the more stimulating its effect on the nervous system. And of course there's also caffeine, North Americans' second-favorite drug next to refined sugar. By way of stimulation, fractionalized foods and caffeinated beverages boost energy nearly immediately. But within only a few hours, that energy will be gone. It is a short-term, unsustainable solution to the symptom of our energy debt. Obtaining energy by way of stimulation is like shopping with a credit card. You get something you desire now, but you will still have to pay eventually. The bill will come. And with that bill comes incurred biological interest: fatigue. Again.

To deal with this second wave of weariness, we tend to rely on additional stimulation, which in turn delays the moment when we pay off our tab. But the longer we put off payment, the greater the debt we accumulate. To continue our credit card analogy, to simply continue to summon energy by way of stimulation is like paying off one credit card with another. All the while, the interest is mounting.

Stimulation is a bad substitute for nourishment for another reason: it prompts the adrenal glands to produce the stress hormone cortisol. Elevated cortisol is linked to inflammation, which is a concern for the athlete (and for anyone who appreciates fluid movement). Higher levels of cortisol also weaken cellular tissue, lower immune response, increase the risk of disease, cause degeneration of body tissue, reduce sleep quality, and are a catalyst for the accumulation of body fat. As if that weren't enough, chronic elevated levels of cortisol reduce the effectiveness of exercise, activity that normally helps to keep cortisol in check. Excessive cortisol levels can actually break down muscle tissue, as well as prevent the action of other hormones that build muscle. As a result, not only do muscles become more difficult to tone but strength is likely to decline rather than increase.

Not surprisingly, if we keep on overstimulating our overstressed body without addressing the real problem behind our fatigue, things only get worse. The severity of the symptoms of stress increase so that our health declines little by little. We put ourselves at greater risk for serious disease.

Common symptoms of adrenal fatigue are increased appetite, followed by cravings, commonly for starchy, refined foods; difficulty sleeping; irritability; mental fog; lack of motivation; body fat gain; lean muscle loss; visible signs of premature aging; and sickness. If this cycle of chronically elevated cortisol levels is allowed to continue, tissue degeneration, depression, chronic fatigue syndrome, and even diseases such as cancer can develop.

In contrast, when we use nutrient-dense whole food rather than fleeting pick-me-ups as our source of energy, our adrenals will not be stimulated, and, simultaneously, our sustainable energy level will rise because of the acquired nutrients. Energy derived from good nutrition—cost-free energy—does not take a toll on the adrenal glands and so doesn't need to be stoked with stimulating substances. In fact, one characteristic of wellness is a ready supply of natural energy that doesn't rely on adrenal stimulation. People who are truly well have boundless energy with no need for stimulants such as caffeine or refined sugar.

"Energy derived from good nutrition—cost-free energy—does not take a toll on the adrenal glands and so doesn't need to be stoked with stimulating substances."

A cornerstone of my dietary philosophy is to break dependency on adrenal stimulation. As you might expect, we accomplish this by basing our diet on—not just supplementing with—nutrient-dense whole foods. This diet, along with proper rest through efficient sleep (efficient because of our reduced stress, thanks to nutrient-dense food), will address the cause of the problem, not just the symptoms of nutritional shortfalls.

Here's a rough visual representation of how most of the recipes will combine to round out a day's worth of eating, Thrive Diet style.

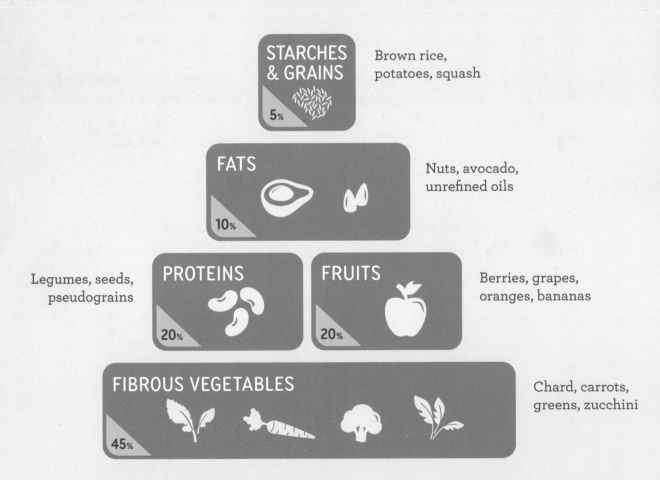

STARCHES & GRAINS — Brown rice, potatoes, squash — 5%

FATS — Nuts, avocado, unrefined oils — 10%

PROTEINS — Legumes, seeds, pseudograins — 20%

FRUITS — Berries, grapes, oranges, bananas — 20%

FIBROUS VEGETABLES — Chard, carrots, greens, zucchini — 45%

Thrive Energy Lab

Five years ago, I received an email from a fellow named Jonnie Karan, who lives in Waterloo, Ontario. Over the course of several heartfelt and chilling paragraphs, he recounted his extremely personal struggle with debilitating sickness. Jonnie told me that he had conquered his health issue and was now not only over his illness but in fact "Thriving." He credited my book *The Thrive Diet* with helping him to view and consume food in a completely different way, a shift that had resulted in his remarkable health turnaround. He concluded by saying that he needed to talk with me. He didn't say why, but insisted it was important. He included his number. I made the call.

In a shaky voice, as though he hadn't spoken in days, he said, "You have no idea how much your book has changed my life, mate. I hope you don't mind, but I had to share with others what your book has done for me. I'm a chef and thought I knew about food. But what I learned about food from your book—I'd feel selfish having this knowledge and not passing it on to others, to help them as it's helped me. So I designed and created a juice bar, modeled after your book. Naturally, I called it Thrive." There was a pause. "I built it in honor of your work and the impact it's had on my life. I hope you don't mind. Would you like to see it? I'd love to show you what we've done. I think you'd be very proud."

Wow. Needless to say, I was delighted to hear of the positive effect that clean, plant-based nutrition had had on Jonnie. But for him to have opened a juice bar so others could benefit in the same way he did? I had to meet this guy.

So I flew from one side of the country to the other, where I met Jonnie, who served me an amazing feast. Jonnie's Thrive Juice Bar was definitely built in line with my vision. Trying his food, I was truly shocked not only by his breadth of recipe creation but also by how innovatively he incorporated all the *Thrive Diet* principles. The flavors and textures of his food were remarkable. I'd always developed recipes with purpose—to serve a function—but Jonnie had added his culinary expertise while maintaining the nutritional intention of the food. In addition, Jonnie created some of the best Vega smoothies I've ever tried. It was truly a case of function meets culinary wizardry.

That was all it took. Jonnie and I became partners, along with others, to create the Thrive Energy Lab. The team at Thrive Energy Lab truly believes that, in tandem with education, there needs to be ease of accessibility. Eating well should never be hard. Our intention is to make mindful, purpose-driven food accessible to all. From day one we shared this common vision, and we would achieve our goal by spreading Thrive Energy Lab restaurants across Canada and eventually into the United States. And that naturally led me to the idea of writing the *Thrive Energy Cookbook* that would allow anyone to reap the benefits of functional, plant-based nutrition.

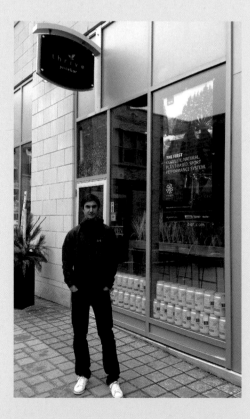

Thrive Energy Cookbook

Inside you'll find 150 Thrive Energy chef-created recipes that are based on the Thrive Diet philosophy and were incubated and tested at Thrive Energy Lab. Complementary flavors and textures have been combined with functional, health-boosting clean, plant-based ingredients to deliver premium recipes that taste as good as they will make you feel and perform. The recipes vary from those that are easy to make at home to those that will require slightly more time and effort, but cooking them is enjoyable, and the flavor and functional benefits make the extra investment well worth it.

From the simplicity of the make-in-minutes, nutrient-packed smoothies and the On-the-Go Breakfast (page 44) with its sprouted bagel, tomato, avocado, and sprouts, to the more complex homemade Cheddar Cashew Cheese (page 24) that needs time to age, you will find plenty of variety in these recipes. Most ingredients can easily be found in your local grocery store, including quinoa and non-dairy milk and cheese. Whenever possible, I've included basic substitutions, but if you're having trouble finding an ingredient, try your local health food or bulk food stores, Whole Foods or Nutshell (in Canada only), or online retailers such as Bob's Red Mill.

Thrive Energy Recipes

The recipes in *Thrive Energy Cookbook* are functional, which means that each ingredient has a nutritional purpose. That's first and foremost. But I've also included some transitional recipes to help those new to this way of eating make the switch as seamlessly as possible. Recipes that I consider to be transitional usually contain a few more traditional ingredients. For example, instead of sweetening with a date, a transition recipe may call for cane sugar. The transition to cleaner ingredients will take a bit of time. But that's okay, because allowing for that transition period means that a new way of eating is much more likely to become habit. These recipes are the ideal starting point.

You'll notice that I don't specify organic ingredients in the recipes. This is simply because, when given the choice, organically grown is the preference for all ingredients. Grown without the use of synthetically produced herbicides or pesticides, organic food by definition cannot have been genetically modified either.

In recipes that call for Medjool dates, you can use either dried or fresh, unless otherwise specified.

In recipes that call for nut milks such as almond milk, you can use rice milk if you have a nut allergy. In recipes that call for filtered water, feel free to use purified water.

I've included the following icons to give more health and nutritional information about each recipe:

T Transition

Indicates recipes designed for those who are accustomed to a more traditional way of eating. These recipes serve as the bridge, helping less healthy eaters transition to the Thrive Diet. The taste profile is in between standard and healthier, allowing the transition to take place without a sudden change. Since this approach eases you into the Thrive way of eating, it dramatically increases the chances of Thrive becoming a lifestyle as opposed to a short-term diet. If you are already a clean eater and accustomed to plant-based whole foods, you may choose to skip these recipes.

R Raw

No ingredient, nor the recipe as a whole, has been heated above 118°F (48°C), and the dish can therefore be considered raw. Not exceeding this temperature keeps enzymes intact, so it makes sense to include raw food in your daily meal plan. Raw food can be as simple as a piece of fruit, or elaborate, such as raw desserts.

GF **Gluten-Free (or recipe includes gluten-free option)** ....

Gluten is the protein found in wheat. It is not inherently bad, but many people do have sensitivities to it and find that it causes digestive issues. Those with celiac disease, which is on the rise, have to avoid gluten altogether.

PR **Protein-Rich** ....

Many people who begin a plant-based diet are concerned that they won't get enough protein. When eating a plant-based whole food diet, lack of protein will not be an issue. However, if you are seeking extra protein, look for this icon.

 Super Nutrient-Dense ....

All the recipes in this book are nutrient-dense, but some stand above the rest and are indicated by this icon. Nutrient density is simply a ratio: number of calories in relation to micronutrient levels (vitamins, minerals, antioxidants, phytochemicals). The goal is to consume the most amount of nutrition (micronutrients) while taking in the fewest calories. The greater the nutrient density, the more filling the food will be while still remaining light in the calorie department. If you're looking to get lean or stay lean, make sure you eat super-nutrient-dense foods several times a day.

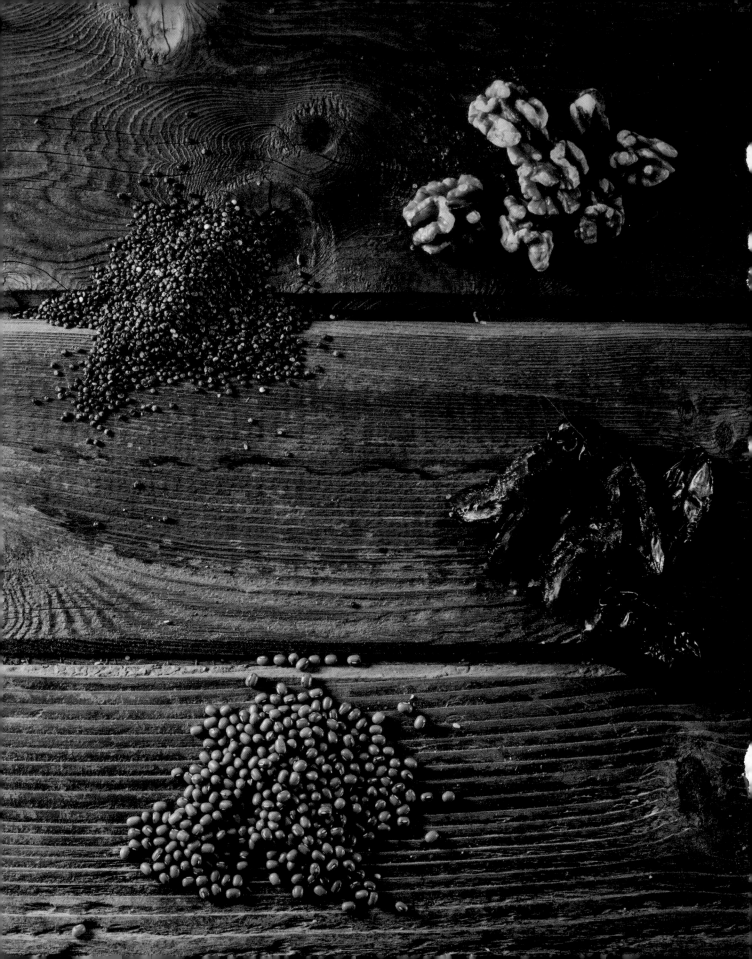

THRIVE ENERGY PANTRY

The staples for most of the recipes in this book are found in the Thrive Diet pyramid on page xxiv. Although some of the foods central to this way of clean, functional eating are not common in a typical North American diet, most of these ingredients can be found in more progressive grocery stores, many bulk food stores, and almost certainly health food stores.

Vegetables

Fibrous vegetables

Fibrous vegetables are the base of the Thrive Diet pyramid, as well as the base of any filling nutrient-dense eating plan. They include

- Asparagus
- Beets
- Bok choy
- Brussels sprouts
- Carrots
- Celery
- Cucumbers
- Daikon
- Green beans
- Green peas
- Onions
- Sugar snap peas
- Squash
- Tomatoes
- Watercress
- Zucchini

Leafy greens

Dark green leafy vegetables are nutrient-dense and a rich source of chlorophyll, important in offsetting stress by alkalizing the body. Chlorophyll also cleanses and oxygenates the blood, making it an essential "modern world" food. Having more oxygen available in the blood reduces fatigue and enhances endurance, so these are great additions to your diet if you are physically active. The consumption of chlorophyll-rich leafy green vegetables, especially raw, combined with moderate exercise is the best way to create a biologically younger body. All leafy greens are healthful and great additions to meals or blended into shakes.

- Beet greens
- Butter lettuce
- Collards
- Dandelion greens
- Dinosaur kale
- Mustard greens
- Red leaf lettuce
- Romaine lettuce
- Spinach
- Swiss chard

Sea vegetables

Sea vegetables, often referred to as seaweed and less commonly as wild ocean plants, have been a staple of many coastal civilizations for thousands of years. Most notably, Asian cultures have long embraced sea vegetables as an important part of their diet.

Sea vegetables are among the most nutritionally dense foods available. Containing about ten times the calcium of cow's milk and several times more iron than red meat, sea vegetables are easily digestible, chlorophyll-rich, and alkaline-forming. Packed with minerals, sea vegetables are the richest known source of naturally occurring electrolytes. Electrolytes allow our cells to stay hydrated longer, thereby improving endurance—of particular significance for active people—so it's important that we get an adequate amount from our diet.

Listed below are the different types of sea vegetables. Dulse is truly the perfect mineral balance in a natural form; it's a superior source of the minerals and trace elements we need daily for optimal health.

- Agar
- Arame
- Dulse
- Kelp
- Kombu
- Nori
- Wakame

Fruits

Fruits frequently used in this cookbook, my favorites, and those I recommend to include in your diet are

- Apples
- Apricots
- Bananas
- Berries (blackberries, blueberries, cranberries, raspberries, strawberries)
- Cherries
- Dates, Medjool
- Dragon fruit
- Figs
- Grapefruit
- Grapes
- Kiwifruit
- Mangoes
- Melons (cantaloupe, honeydew, watermelon)
- Nectarines
- Oranges
- Papayas
- Peaches
- Pears
- Pineapples
- Plums
- Pomegranates

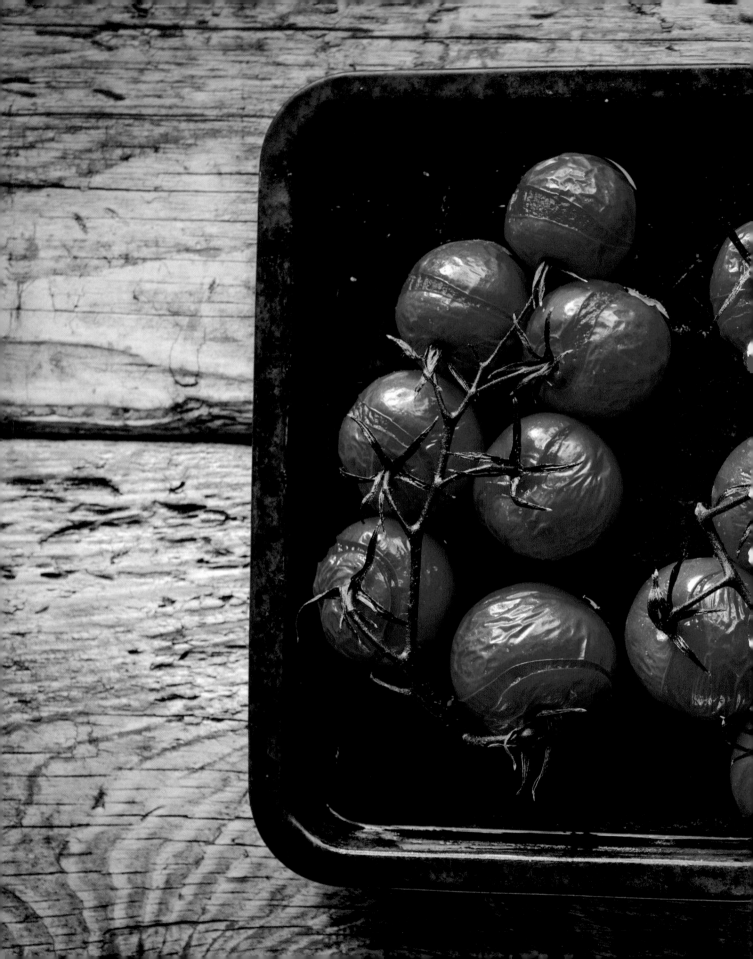

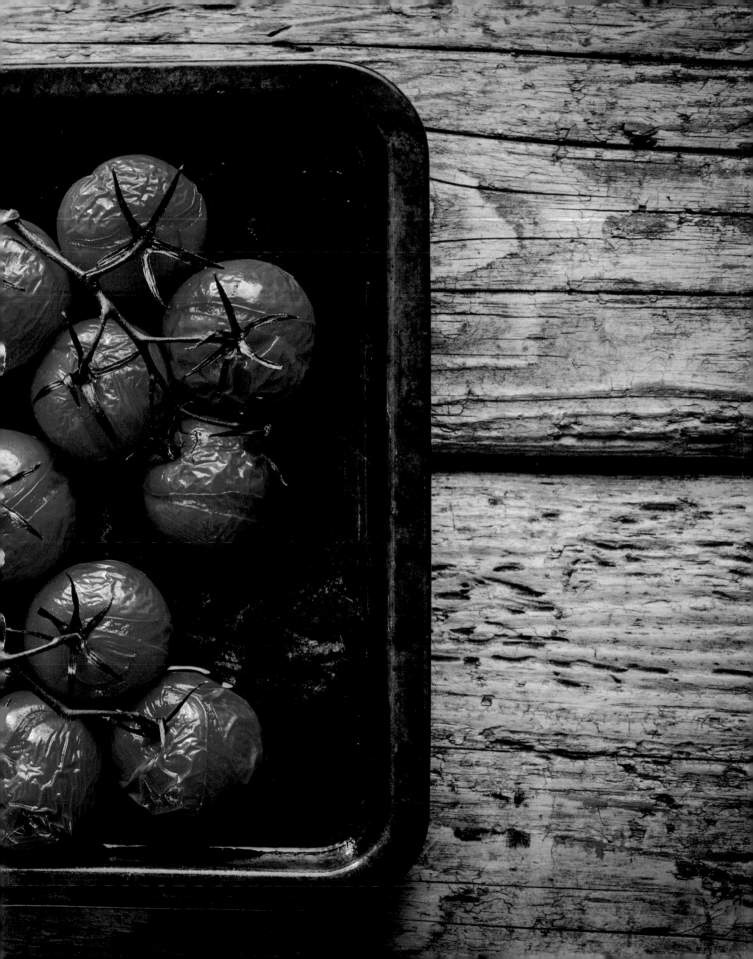

Legumes

Legumes are a family of plants that have pods containing small seeds. Lentils, peas, and beans are all in the legume family. Lentils and split peas are popular for the simple reason that they don't need to be soaked before cooking.

Legumes in general have an excellent nutritional profile, high in protein, fiber, and many vitamins and minerals. I include a variety of legumes in my regular diet. Peas, and in particular yellow peas, have an exceptional amino acid profile. Also rich in B vitamins and potassium, yellow peas are an excellent addition to your diet, especially if you are active.

Although some people avoid legumes because of their gas-producing reputation, legumes are no more a culprit than any other food, as long as they are prepared properly. After you soak beans and shelled peas before cooking them, be sure to rinse them in fresh water. Rinse them again in fresh water after cooking. The water they soak and cook in will absorb some of the indigestible sugars that cause gas; rinsing helps to improve their digestibility and minimize gas production. Another way to improve legumes' digestibility is to add seaweed to the pot when cooking them, to release the gas. A short strip of seaweed is enough for a medium pot.

As with all fiber-rich foods, legumes should be introduced slowly into the diet to allow time for the digestive system to adapt. Gradually increasing the amount of legumes you eat each day will ensure a smooth transition to a clean Thrive Diet. I recommend these legumes for their nutritional value and taste:

Beans
- Adzuki
- Black
- Chickpeas (garbanzo beans)
- Fava
- Kidney
- Navy
- Pinto

Lentils
- Brown
- Green
- Red

Peas
- Black-eyed
- Green, split
- Yellow, split

Seeds

Flaxseed

Flaxseeds contain high levels of omega-3, an essential fatty acid. Omega-3 and omega-6 are considered "essential" because the body cannot produce them. Omega-6 is easy to obtain in a healthy diet; it is prevalent in many nuts, seeds, and vegetable oils. In contrast, omega-3 is rare in the plant kingdom, although hemp and walnuts contain some. Flaxseed, however, is the most abundant source of omega-3 (57 percent of its total fat), making it a vital addition to the vegetarian or vegan diet and very important to athletes. Aside from its ability to help reduce inflammation caused by movement, omega-3 plays an integral part in the metabolism of fat. A diet with a daily dose of 10 grams (about 1 tbsp/15 mL) of ground whole flaxseeds will allow the body to more efficiently burn body fat as fuel.

Hemp seeds

Hemp's protein is complete protein, containing all ten essential amino acids that must be obtained through diet since the body doesn't produce them. This makes hemp superior to many other sources of protein. Hemp's full spectrum of essential amino acids offers a clear benefit especially if you are active. Its amino acid profile helps boost the body's immune system and its anti-inflammatory properties speed recovery. A high-quality complete protein such as hemp is instrumental not only in muscle and tissue regeneration but also in fat metabolism.

I find hemp protein to be more easily digested than all other proteins I've tried. Since hemp protein is raw, its naturally occurring digestive enzymes remain intact, allowing the body to utilize it with the greatest of ease, reducing digestive strain. Because of its easy digestibility and absorption, hemp protein is a good replacement for other proteins. In fact, you will need to consume less protein if you choose a high-quality protein like hemp: quality, not quantity, is paramount.

Protein, once ingested, instigates the release of a hormone that enables the body to more easily use its fat reserves, which in turn improves endurance and facilitates loss of body fat. Because hemp foods are raw, they maintain their naturally high level of vitamins, high-quality balanced fats, antioxidants, and alkaline-forming chlorophyll.

Freshness is particularly important when selecting hemp foods, including hemp oil, hemp seeds, and hemp protein powder. A deep green color, pleasant smell, and sweet, nutty taste are indications of a recent harvest. As with any crop, be sure to choose hemp that has been grown without the use of herbicides or pesticides.

Pumpkin seeds

Pumpkin seeds are rich in iron, a nutrient some people have trouble getting enough of, especially if they don't eat red meat. Anemia, a shortage of red blood cells in the body, is commonly caused by low dietary iron or by strenuous exercise. The more active you are, the more dietary iron you need. I always keep raw pumpkin seeds on hand, sprinkling them on many of my meals.

Sesame seeds

Sesame seeds are an excellent, easily absorbable source of calcium. Calcium is in part responsible for muscle contractions, so it's important for those who are active, especially if you live in a warm climate. Calcium is also key to maintaining good bone and teeth health.

Sunflower seeds

About 22 percent protein, sunflower seeds offer a good amount of dietary substance. Rich in trace minerals and several vitamins important for good health, they are a food worthy of regular consumption. Sunflower seeds are quite high in vitamin E and are antioxidant-rich. Also, raw sunflower seeds can be used in place of almonds for making milk, on a one-to-one ratio.

Pseudograins

Pseudograins are actually seeds, though they are commonly referred to as grains. Pseudograins don't contain gluten, which makes them easily digestible, alkaline-forming, and suitable for celiacs and those who are gluten-intolerant.

Amaranth

With its nutty flavor and high nutrition density, amaranth is one of my favorite pseudograins. Amaranth is quite high in calcium, iron, potassium, phosphorus, and vitamins A and C. About 17 percent protein, amaranth is particularly rich in lysine, an elusive essential amino acid. Lysine is important for the absorption of calcium from the digestive tract, but it can be difficult to find in plant-based foods, which qualifies amaranth as a worthy addition to a diet for optimum nutrition. In addition, ounce for ounce, amaranth has twice the calcium of cow's milk. Amaranth consists of about 8 percent fatty acids, found mostly in its germ. Within those fats is a valuable form of vitamin E known as tocotrienol, a powerful antioxidant. Amaranth is easy on the digestive system and as such is considered a high-net-gain food.

With about three times the fiber of wheat flour and almost five times the iron, including amaranth flour in recipes for baked foods is an easy way to boost nutritional value. But because of its strong, sweet flavor, it is best used as a secondary flour, combined with a primary flour such as spelt or kamut. Amaranth flour also has a gummy texture. Combining it with fluffier grain or seed flours, such as spelt or buckwheat, is a good way to offset this.

Preparation: Cook like rice, at a 1:3 amaranth-to-water ratio, for about 25 minutes.

Buckwheat

Despite its name, buckwheat is not wheat, nor is it even in the wheat family. In fact, buckwheat is related to rhubarb. Containing eight essential amino acids, including high amounts of the often elusive tryptophan, buckwheat is considered a good-quality source of protein. Since tryptophan is a precursor for serotonin (which means serotonin is formed from tryptophan), having an adequate amount of it in your diet is important to help enhance your mood and mental clarity. Buckwheat is very high in manganese and quite high in vitamins B and E; it also provides calcium.

Because of its mild flavor, buckwheat is easily overwhelmed by the foods it accompanies. The amino acid profile of buckwheat flour nicely complements that of quinoa flour when the two are combined. When buying, be sure to select the unroasted form. Roasted buckwheat, also known as kasha, is an east European staple. Roasted buckwheat cannot be sprouted and is less versatile in recipes.

Preparation: Cook like rice, at a 1:3 buckwheat-to-water ratio, for about 20 minutes.

Quinoa

With a light, fluffy texture and mild earthy taste, quinoa balances the texture of other, heavier grains when combined with them. Nutritionally similar to amaranth, quinoa is about 20 percent protein; it is high in lysine and is a good source of iron and potassium. High levels of B vitamins, in part responsible for the conversion of carbohydrate into energy, are also found in quinoa.

Quinoa is naturally coated in a bitter resin called saponin, thought to have evolved to deter birds and insects from eating the seed. Most of the saponin will have been removed before the quinoa is shipped to the store, but there will likely be a powdery residue. To make quinoa palatable, it must be thoroughly rinsed to remove any remaining saponin.

Preparation: Cook like rice, at a 1:2 quinoa-to-water ratio, for about 15 minutes.

Wild rice

Wild rice is an aquatic grass seed rather than a true rice. High in B vitamins and the amino acid lysine, wild rice is much more nutritious than traditional grains. Native to the northern regions of the Canadian prairie provinces, wild rice is seldom treated with pesticides since it thrives without them. (It is also grown as a domesticated crop in Minnesota and California.) Wild rice has a distinct full-bodied flavor and slightly chewy texture that complements many meals.

Preparation: Cook like rice, at a 1:2 wild rice-to-water ratio, for about 30 minutes.

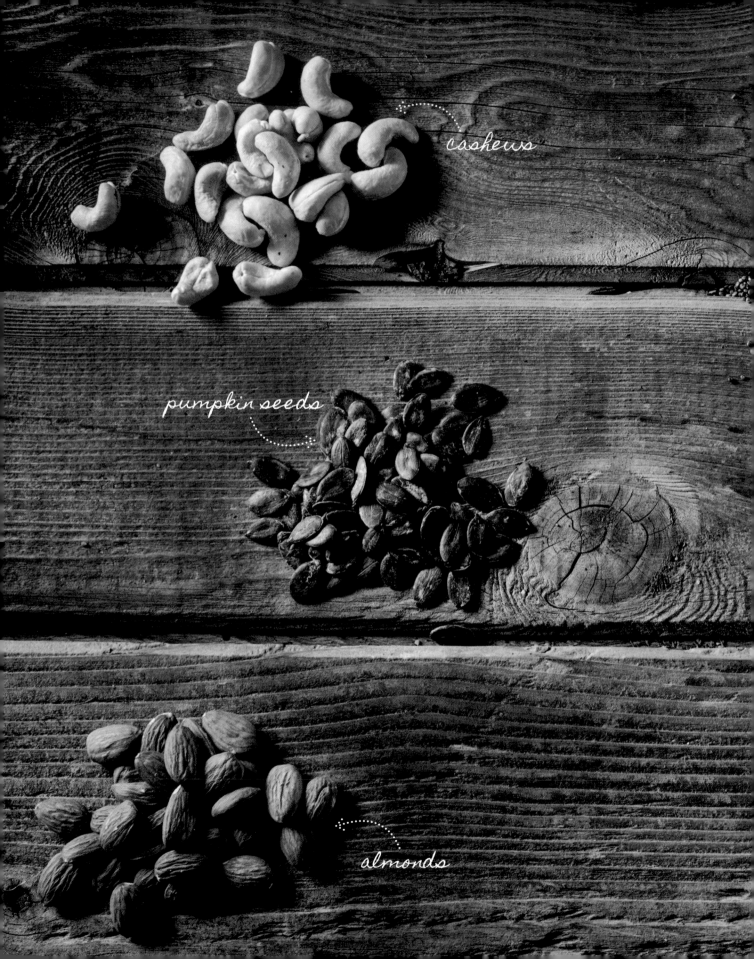

cashews

pumpkin seeds

almonds

walnuts

quinoa

Medjool dates

mung beans

Starches & Grains

Starchy vegetables

Starchy vegetables are an important part of clean eating and are part of the Thrive philosophy, but only small amounts are needed. Good choices include

- New potatoes
- Parsnips
- Pumpkin
- Squash
- Sweet potatoes
- Turnips
- Yams

Brown rice

Brown rice isn't processed as extensively as white rice, making it nutritionally superior to its white counterpart. Since its bran layer isn't removed, brown rice retains its nutritional value. Brown rice is very high in manganese and contains large amounts of selenium and magnesium. It is a good source of B vitamins as well.

   Preparation: Cook like white rice, at a 1:2 rice-to-water ratio, for about 45 minutes.

Millet

Millet is one of the most easily digested grains, and it's gluten-free. It's also probably the most versatile grain. Millet can be either creamy or fluffy, depending on how long it is cooked. High in B vitamins, magnesium, and the essential amino acid tryptophan, millet is nutritionally dense and complements many meals. Millet flour has a mild taste, and it absorbs the flavor of whatever it is combined with.

   Preparation: Cook like rice, at a 1:3 millet-to-water ratio, for about 35 minutes. It can also be sprouted.

Spelt

Spelt is rich in energy-producing B vitamins and has 30 percent more protein than standard whole wheat. Spelt does contain gluten but in considerably smaller quantities than whole wheat. Because of its gluten content, spelt flour can be used to bind other grain and seed flours in baking. For this reason, and because spelt takes longer than most grains to prepare, spelt flour is the most useful form of this grain. Spelt has a mild, slightly nutty flavor.

   Preparation: Soak overnight, then cook like rice, at a 1:3 spelt-to-water ratio, for about 1 hour. It can also be sprouted.

Teff

Teff is a delicious mineral-rich grain. Along with its large amounts of calcium, magnesium, boron, copper, phosphorus, and zinc, teff has about twice as much iron as whole wheat. This tiny grain becomes creamy when cooked; reduce cooking time for a slightly crunchy texture. Teff has a slight molasses taste, adding flavor when combined with other grain and seed flours.

Preparation: Cook like rice, at a 1:4 teff-to-water ratio, for about 15 minutes. It can also be sprouted.

Oils

Oils come in a wide assortment, each with a distinct taste and its own nutritional value. The key to keeping the flavors in your meals ever changing and your diet's nutrient value diverse is using various oils. (By "diverse" I mean that each meal or snack will offer nutrients that complement nutrients in other meals. So over the course of the day, all nutrients will be present, but they are not all present in each meal.) In the right amount, high-quality, cold-pressed, unrefined oils are among the healthiest of substances. My favorites are hemp, pumpkin, flaxseed, and, for cooking, coconut. Most oils contain the same nutrients as the plant seed they are derived from, just highly concentrated.

Not all oils are equal. Low-quality manufactured oil is one of the most damaging foods that can be consumed, eclipsing even refined carbohydrate. Many cheaper store-bought baked or fried products, such as muffins, chips, and cakes, contain trans fat, a near-poisonous substance unusable by the body. Trans fat, also known as trans-fatty acid, is added to many mass-produced commercial products to extend their shelf life, improve moisture content, and enhance flavor.

It's important to know which oils can be heated safely and which are best consumed raw. I never fry with hemp, flaxseed, or pumpkin seed oil because of their low burning (or smoke) point—the temperature at which an oil becomes molecularly damaged. Exceeding the burning point can convert healthy oils into trans-fatty acids. When baking with ingredients that contain fatty acids, such as flaxseed and other milled seeds, it is important that the temperature not exceed 350°F (180°C). I rarely bake anything at temperatures above 300°F (150°C), to ensure that the fatty acids retain their nutritional value. For stir-frying, where the temperature is likely to exceed 350°F (180°C), I use only coconut oil.

Coconut oil

Coconut oil is produced by pressing the meat of the coconut. This is the only fat I use for frying. Solid at room temperature, coconut oil can be heated to a high temperature without converting to a trans fat. Surprisingly, coconut oil does not have a strong coconut taste, and it has almost no smell. When used in cooking, any remaining hint of the coconut taste disappears, making this a versatile oil. Coconut oil is rich in medium-chain triglycerides, or MCTs. MCTs are unique in that they are a form of saturated fat yet have several health benefits. The body utilizes them differently than fat that does not contain MCTs. Their digestion is nearly effortless. In fact, within moments of MCTs being consumed, the liver converts them to energy.

Extra-virgin olive oil

"Extra-virgin" means that the oil is from the first pressing of the olive. The subsequent pressing is referred to as virgin, and the one after that produces regular olive oil. With a light taste and color, extra-virgin olive oil is a healthy addition to sauces, dips, and dressings. Although extra-virgin olive oil is a healthful oil, it delivers only minimal amounts of omega-3.

Flaxseed oil

Flaxseed oil is obtained by pressing flaxseed. Milder in taste than hemp and pumpkin seed oils, flaxseed oil contains the highest amount of omega-3 in comparison to omega-6, at a 5:1 ratio.

Hemp oil

Obtained by pressing hemp seed, hemp oil is one of the healthiest oils available. Dark green with a smooth, creamy texture and a mild nutty flavor, hemp oil is an excellent base for salad dressings. Hemp oil is unique in that it has the ideal ratio of omega-6 and omega-3 fatty acids.

Pumpkin seed oil

Pumpkin seed oil is a deep green color with a hint of dark red. With a distinct robust flavor, pumpkin seed oil is packed with essential fatty acids and has been linked to improved prostate health.

Nuts

Almonds

The almond is one of the most popular nuts in North America. Almonds are resistant to mold in the raw state, making them a perfect nut to soak and eat raw. Particularly high in vitamin B2, fiber, and antioxidants, almonds have one of the highest nutrient levels of all nuts. That, combined with their high level of digestibility, especially when soaked, makes them a worthy addition to your diet. Although almonds don't need to be soaked, soaking does make them more nutritious—in this pre-sprouting state, their vitamin levels increase and the enzyme inhibitors are removed, making them even more efficiently digested. I've included a simple recipe for almond milk (page 23) that can be used in place of any store-bought milk. If you have a nut allergy, use rice milk instead.

Macadamia nuts

Macadamia nuts contain omega-7 and omega-9 fatty acids. While these are nonessential fatty acids, meaning the body produces them, their inclusion in the diet has been linked to positive health benefits. Blending soaked macadamia nuts results in a creamy spread that makes for a healthy alternative to butter or margarine. Although soaked macadamia nuts are recommended for any of my recipes calling for macadamia nuts, they don't need to be soaked if you're short of time or unprepared.

Walnuts

Walnuts are rich in B vitamins and possess a unique amino acid profile. Also rich in potassium and magnesium, walnuts can help maintain adequate electrolyte levels in the body, prolonging hydration. As with almonds and macadamia nuts, soaking improves their nutrition and digestibility. Walnuts complement many meals and snacks.

Other nuts

The nuts listed below all offer high levels of nutrition in a compact form. These nuts can be substituted for the more common nuts such as almonds and macadamia. Incorporating a range of nuts into your diet will ensure a greater variety of taste and nutrition.

- Brazil nuts
- Cashew nuts
- Hazelnuts (filberts)
- Pecans
- Pine nuts
- Pistachios

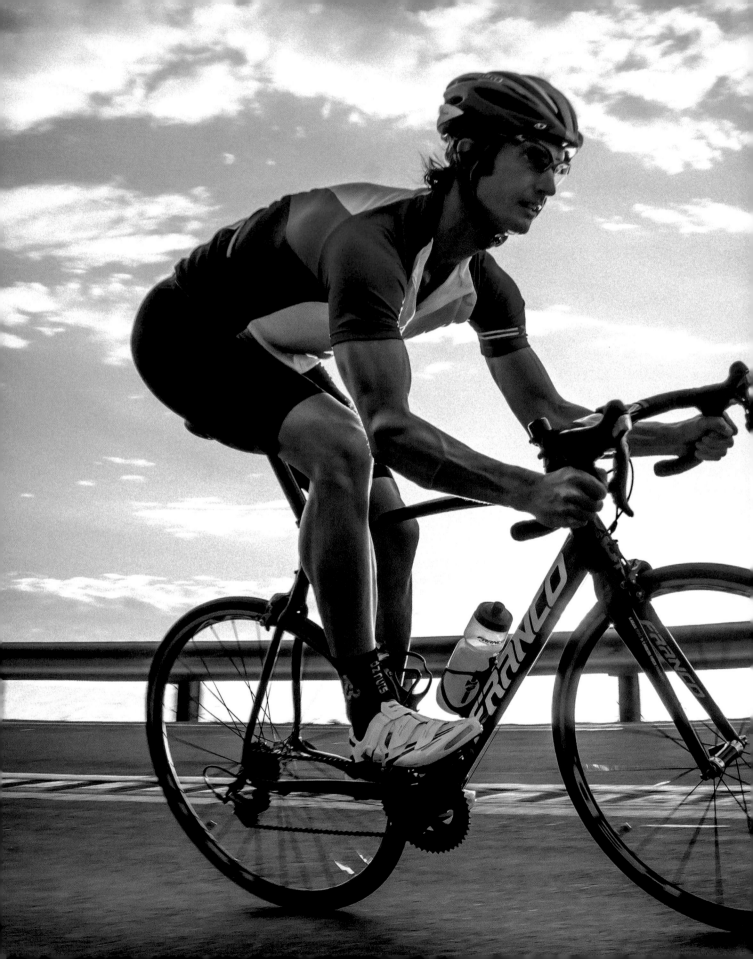

"Take control of your health;
write your future."

Vinegars

Cider vinegar

Apple cider vinegar adds plenty of potassium to sauces and salad dressings. Made from fermented apples, cider vinegar is considered a healthy vinegar, whereas traditional white vinegar is not. It also contains malic acid, which aids digestion.

Balsamic vinegar

As with cider vinegar, balsamic vinegar has an alkalizing effect on the system. Combined with hemp oil or another oil blend, balsamic vinegar makes a good salad dressing base.

Nutritional Yeast

Nutritional yeast is a single-cell fungus grown on molasses. A complete protein and a rich source of B vitamins, nutritional yeast is especially prized for its vitamin B12 content. Vitamin B12 is scarce in the plant kingdom, so nutritional yeast provides a reliable source for those on a plant-based diet. Unlike baking yeast, nutritional yeast in not active, meaning that it does not feed and grow once inside the body. For this reason, those who are advised to avoid yeast (usually meaning active yeast) can almost always tolerate nutritional yeast. Because it melts and has a mild Cheddar cheese flavor, nutritional yeast is a good flavor and nutritional addition to sauces, soups, and salads.

Sweeteners

Stevia

Stevia is an herb that's about thirty times sweeter than sugar, but dried stevia contains no carbohydrates and so has no effect on the body's insulin or blood sugar levels when ingested. It's a natural sugar substitute—and an excellent alternative to manufactured artificial sweeteners—with the added benefit of improving digestion.

Coconut nectar

Derived from the sap of the coconut blossom, coconut nectar is a low-glycemic carbohydrate source that is an ideal endurance fuel. Since it is composed of clean-burning sugar, it also adds a mild sweetness to recipes.

Agave nectar

Most commonly derived from the blue agave plant, agave nectar is a sweet, syrup-like substance that is a clean-burning fuel source. Since it is almost 100 percent sugar, it will cause insulin to rise quickly if it is not consumed with a fat, protein, or fiber source. Therefore, it is best used as a functional ingredient in sport nutrition products such as bars.

Herbs

Below are the herbs that I like to use most. It's always best to use fresh herbs, but it's good to keep dried herbs on hand in your pantry.

- Basil
- Chilies
- Cilantro
- Dill
- Mint
- Oregano
- Parsley
- Thyme

Spices

Along with sea salt, it's good to keep a well-stocked supply of spices you like to use regularly. Here are some of my favorites:

- Black pepper
- Cardamom
- Cayenne
- Cinnamon
- Cloves
- Coriander
- Cumin
- Curry powder
- Nutmeg
- Paprika
- Turmeric

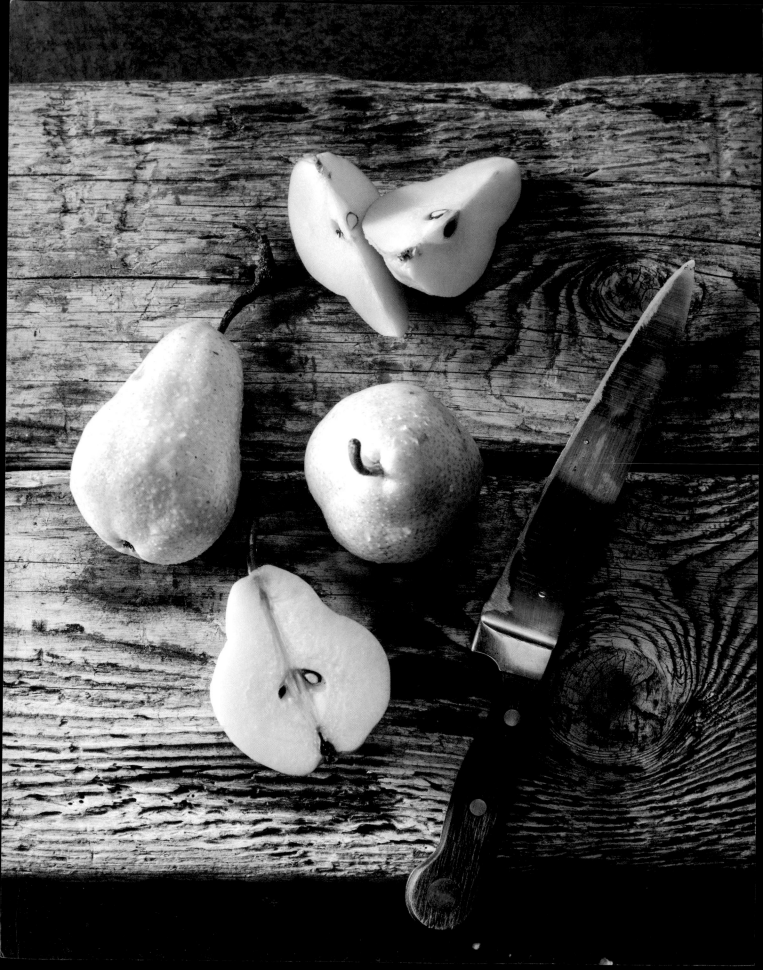

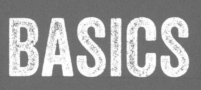

BASICS

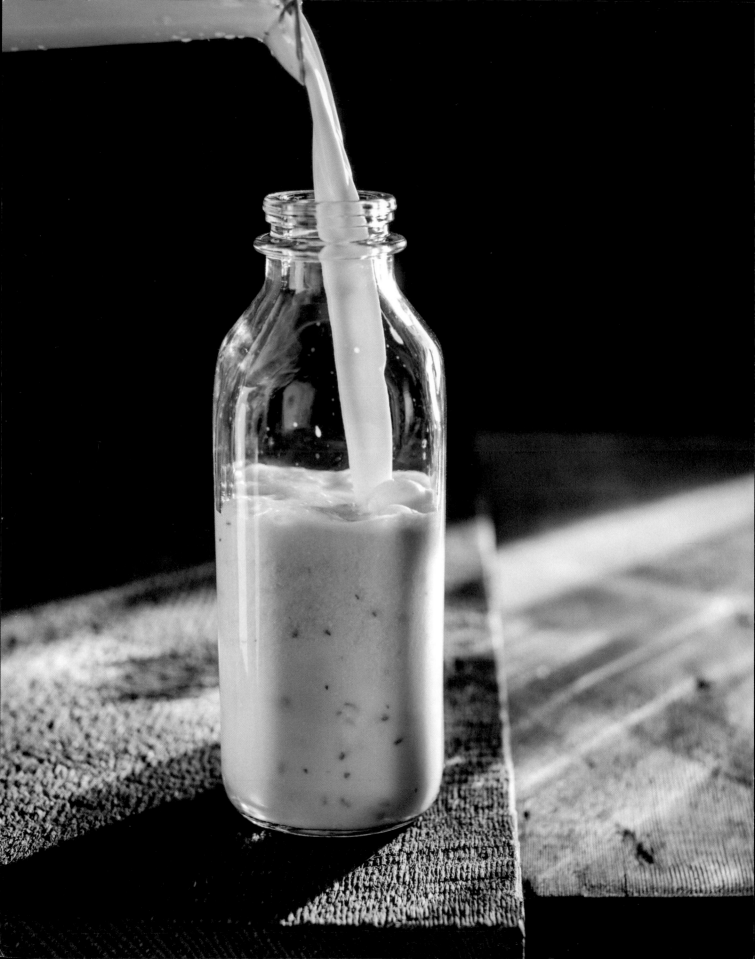

ALMOND MILK

Simple and raw, this versatile nut milk is loaded with nutrition, without the fillers included in some store-bought versions. Store-bought nut milks are also pasteurized, which reduces their nutritional value. Almond milk can be used whenever nut milk is called for in a recipe, and of course it's ideal on cereal. **Makes 4 cups (1 L)**

R Raw   **GF** Gluten-Free   **PR** Protein-Rich

Prep Time: 5 minutes, plus 8 to 10 hours soaking time
Special Equipment: high-speed blender, fine-mesh sieve

Soak the almonds in a bowl of water for 8 to 10 hours. The longer the soak, the creamier the almond milk, up to about 12 hours. Drain and rinse the almonds.

In a blender, combine the soaked almonds, 2 cups (500 mL) of the water, and the date (if using). Blend on low at first, then blend on high for 1 to 2 minutes or until smooth and milky.

Add the remaining 1 cup (250 mL) water and blend for another 20 seconds.

Strain the almond mixture through a fine-mesh sieve into a bowl, then strain again in a nut bag or through cheesecloth, extracting as much liquid as possible. Discard the solids.

Increase sweetness to taste, if desired, by adding another date or coconut nectar. Add salt.

1 cup (250 mL) raw almonds

3 cups (750 mL) water

1 Medjool date, pitted (optional, if you prefer sweeter)

Pinch of sea salt

- Keeps in an unsealed container, refrigerated, for up to 5 days.
- To make chocolate milk, add 2 tsp (10 mL) cacao powder.
- You can use any other raw nuts or seeds, or a combination of several, such as hemp, sunflower, cashew (for the creamiest milk), or walnuts.

CHEDDAR CASHEW CHEESE

This cheese gives a nutrition and flavor boost to any burger. It takes a little time to make, but it is truly a unique and versatile recipe that provides loads of nutrition.
Makes 1 lb (450 g)

R Raw   **GF** Gluten-Free   **PR** Protein-Rich

Prep Time: 5 minutes, plus 6 to 8 hours soaking time
Special Equipment: blender

2 cups (500 mL) raw cashews

⅔ cup (150 mL) nutritional yeast flakes

½ cup (125 mL) rejuvelac (recipe follows)

½ tsp (2 mL) garlic powder

4 tsp (20 mL) brown miso

1 tsp (5 mL) sea salt

2 tbsp (30 mL) agar powder

Soak the cashews in a bowl of filtered water for 6 to 8 hours. Drain the cashews.

Combine the cashews and all of the remaining ingredients except for the agar powder in a blender. Blend until smooth. Transfer the mixture to a glass bowl and cover with cheesecloth. Let sit at room temperature for 24 to 72 hours.

Transfer mixture to a saucepan and stir in agar powder on medium heat. Stir consistently for 3 to 5 minutes until smooth. Transfer cheese to a square glass container to form into a small block. Smooth out the top.

Refrigerate for at least 6 hours or until somewhat firm.

• Keeps, wrapped in plastic wrap and refrigerated, for up to 3 weeks. The longer the cheese ages in the fridge, the sharper it will taste. At the Thrive Energy Lab, we age it for 2 weeks.

REJUVELAC

The magic ingredient needed to make Cheddar Cashew Cheese. Makes 4 cups (1 L)

 R Raw   **GF** Gluten-Free   **SND** Super Nutrient-Dense

Total Time: about 6 days
Special Equipment: medium to large mason jar

In a bowl, soak the quinoa in 2 cups (500 mL) of the filtered water for 8 to 12 hours. Drain quinoa, rinse twice, and transfer to a mason jar. Cover with cheesecloth and let sit at room temperature, rinsing two or three times a day, until the grains start sprouting and little tails appear. This may take 10 to 12 hours.

Add 4 cups (1 L) filtered water. Cover with cheesecloth and let sit for another 2 days.

Strain, discarding the sprouted grains. Store the liquid in the refrigerator. It should smell and taste fresh but should also be cloudy.

1 cup (250 mL) quinoa, soft wheat berries, or buckwheat

6 cups (1.5 L) filtered water

....

- Keeps in a sealed glass jar, refrigerated, for up to 1 week.
- Fermented foods are easily contaminated, so be sure to use clean, disinfected jars and tools.

ALMOND BUTTER

Always good to have on hand, homemade almond butter is a simple, versatile, two-ingredient staple that is full of nutrition. Makes 2 cups (500 mL)

 R Raw   GF Gluten-Free   PR Protein-Rich

Prep Time: 5 minutes • **Special Equipment:** food processor

2 cups (500 mL) raw almonds
Pinch of sea salt

Line a baking sheet with parchment paper and spread out the almonds. Roast at 350°F (180°C) for 6 to 8 minutes.

Let the almonds cool and blend in a food processor for 12 to 15 minutes straight, only stopping to scrape down the walls every few minutes, if needed, until achieving a thick and creamy texture.

Add the sea salt and blend to incorporate.

• Store in a mason jar in the fridge for about 3 weeks.

Variations

Sweet Almond Butter: Add 1 tbsp (15 mL) maple syrup or coconut nectar.

Chocolate Almond Butter: Add 3 tbsp (45 mL) coconut oil and 3 tbsp (45 mL) cacao powder.

Maple Cinnamon Almond Butter: Add 2 tbsp (30 mL) maple syrup and 1 tsp (5 mL) cinnamon.

COCONUT BUTTER

A delicious alternative to traditional butter or margarine, this functional combination of healthy oils can be spread on toasted sprouted bread, melted over freshly steamed vegetables, and even used in baking—substitute the same amount of coconut butter for the traditional butter your recipe calls for.

Makes about 1¼ cups (300 mL)

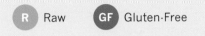 **R** Raw   **GF** Gluten-Free

---

Prep Time: 20 minutes • **Special Equipment:** food processor or blender

In a food processor or blender, process the coconut for 12 to 15 minutes, scraping the sides down every few minutes.

3 cups (750 mL) unsweetened full fat shredded coconut

....

• The blender is quicker, but the food processor makes a better quality butter.
• It will keep in the refrigerator for 2 weeks.

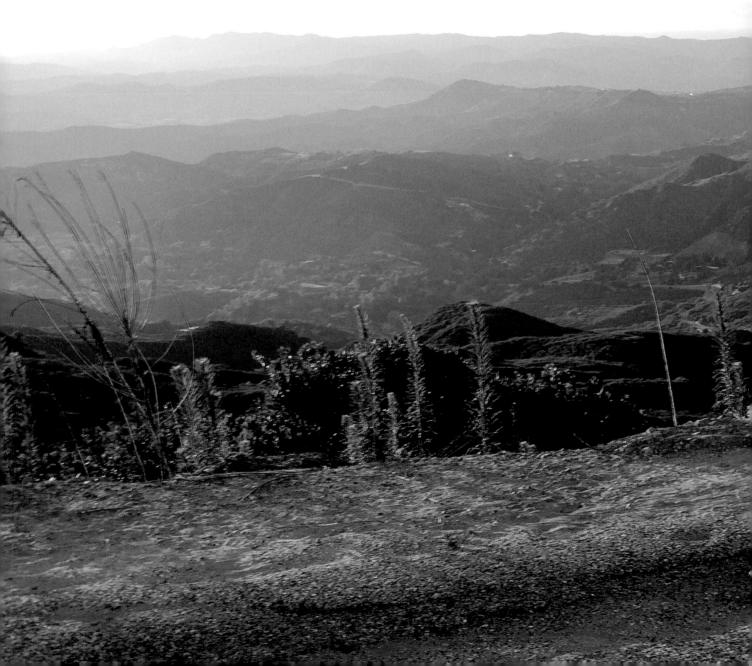

"As close as you can get to perfection is continual improvement."

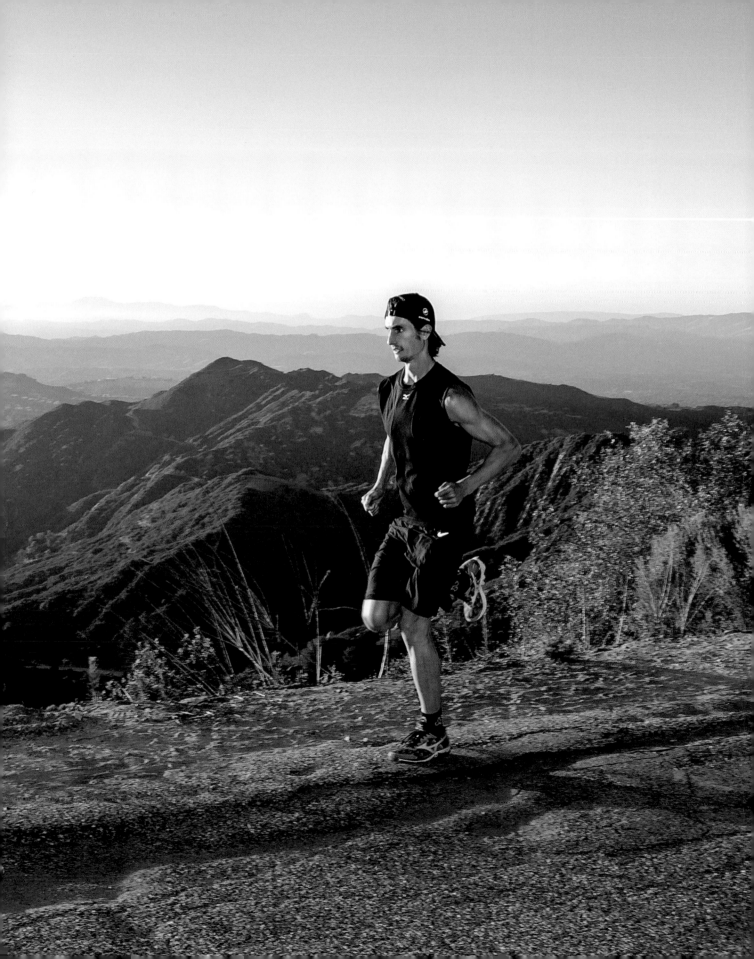

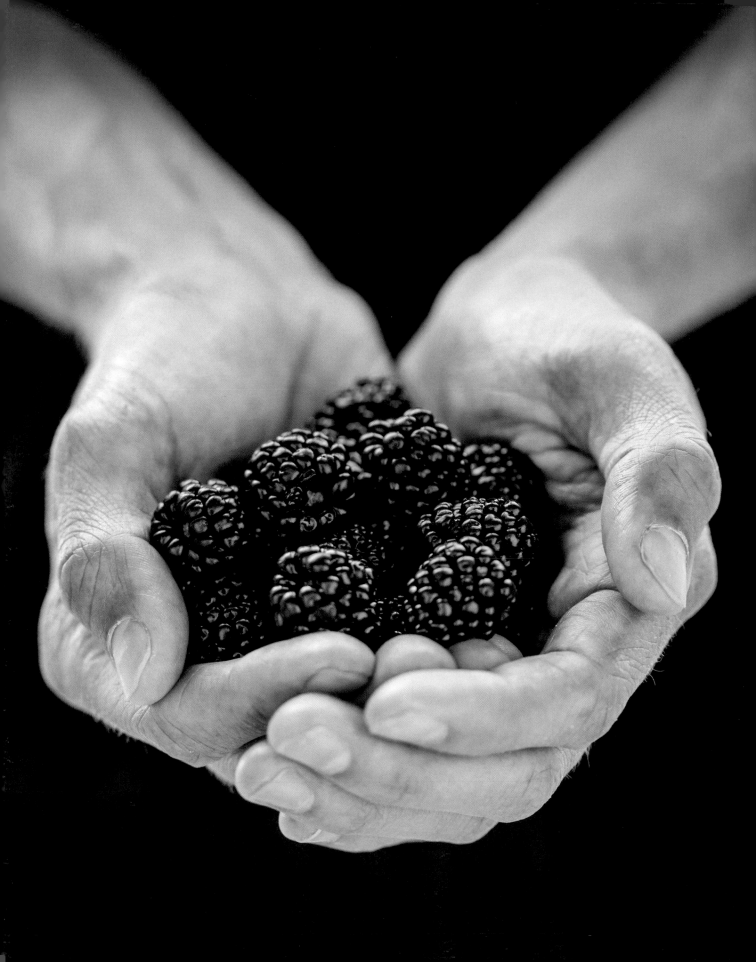

MORNINGS

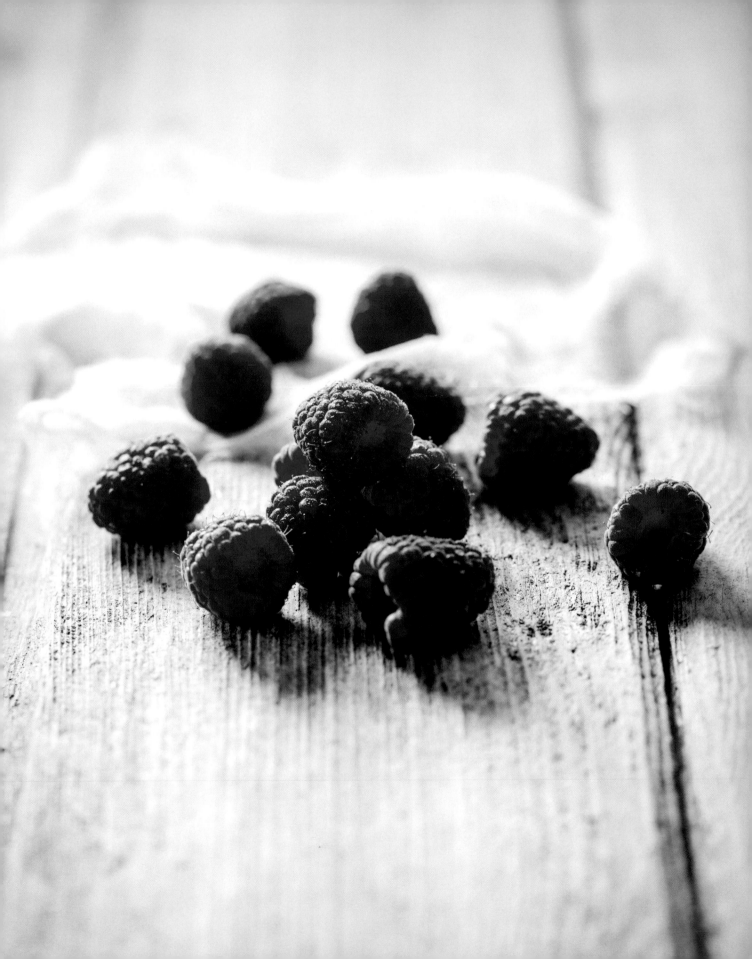

RASPBERRY LEMON YERBA MATE

An invigorating antioxidant-rich kick in the morning, this is an ideal coffee substitute, containing natural caffeine from the phytonutrient-rich yerba mate.

Serves 1/Makes 1¾ cups (425 mL)

 Gluten-Free

Prep Time: 4 minutes

Steep the tea in hot water for 3 to 4 minutes.

Remove the tea bag or strain the loose leaves. Stir in the maple syrup. Add the lemon slices and raspberries. Garnish with fresh mint leaves.

1 yerba mate tea bag (or 1 tsp/5 mL loose tea)

1⅔ cups (400 mL) hot water

1 tsp (5 mL) maple syrup (or stevia if you prefer to keep low carb), or to taste

2 slices lemon

1 handful of frozen or fresh raspberries

2 fresh mint leaves or small sprig, for garnish

CHIA LIME ALOE FRESCA

This exceptionally refreshing drink combines the phytonutrients that chia has become renowned for with the stomach-settling qualities of aloe vera. It's an ideal drink to kick-start your morning and help maintain hydration, and therefore energy, throughout the day. It's especially nice on a warm summer day.

Serves 1/Makes 1¾ cups (425 mL)

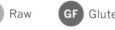 Raw   Gluten-Free   **SND** Super Nutrient-Dense

Prep Time: 10 minutes

1¼ cups (300 mL) filtered water

3 tbsp (45 mL) aloe vera juice

2 tbsp (30 mL) freshly squeezed lime juice

2 tbsp (30 mL) maple syrup (or stevia if you prefer to keep low carb), or to taste

2 tsp (10 mL) chia seeds

In a tall cup, combine the water, aloe vera juice, and lime juice. Stir in the maple syrup. Stir in the chia seeds and let soak until they gelatinize, usually 4 to 5 minutes. Stir while soaking to avoid clumping.

• This drink is awesome cold, so add ice or refrigerate a big batch for friends.

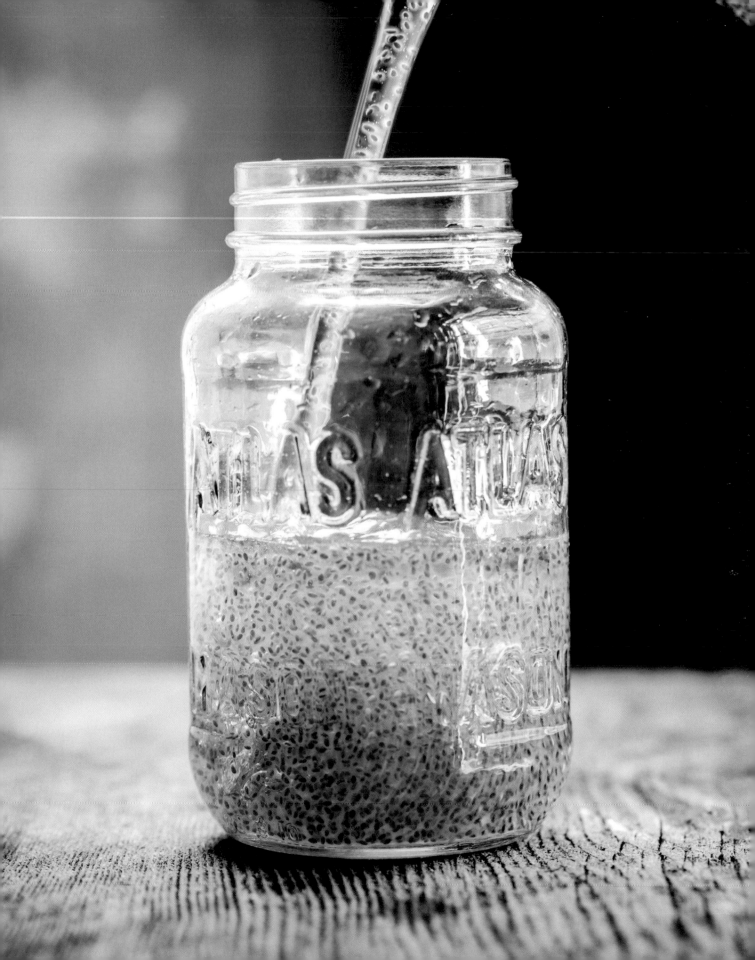

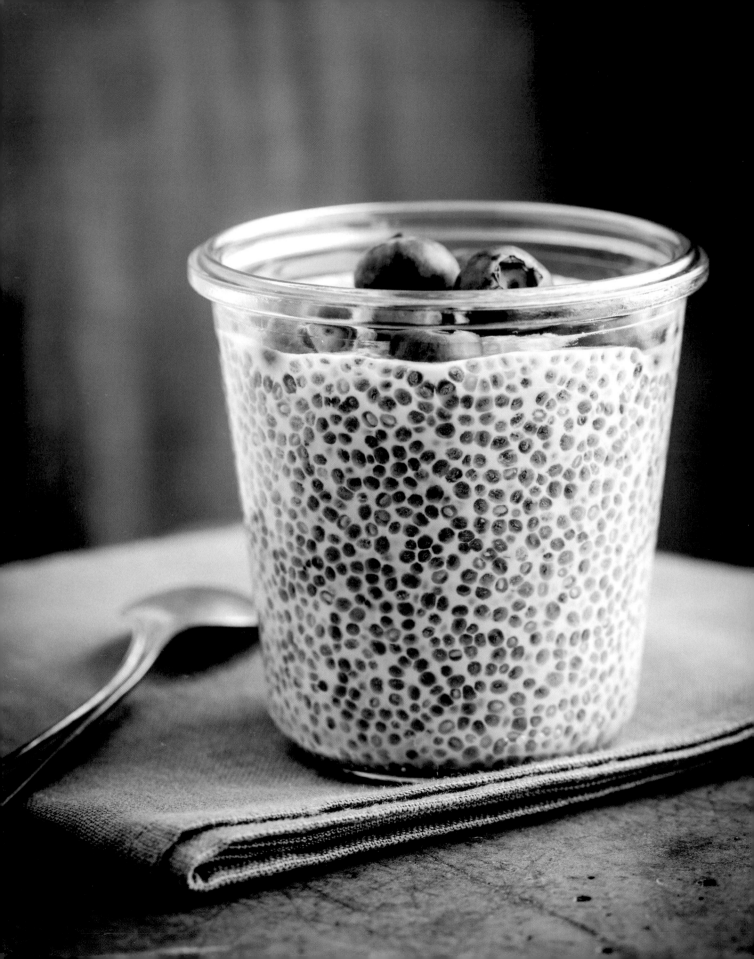

CHIA SEED BLUEBERRY MAPLE PUDDING

Easily digestible and packed with antioxidants, this energizing pudding is a beautiful start to any morning. It's also a great post-workout breakfast option. You can use frozen blueberries in a pinch, but fresh is preferred. Serves 2

 Raw   Gluten-Free   **SND** Super Nutrient-Dense

Prep Time: 5 minutes

In a bowl, add the almond milk, latte spice mix, maple syrup and lastly, the chia seeds.

Let sit for 15 minutes, stirring once or twice.

Garnish with fresh blueberries.

. . . .

• Keeps in an unsealed container, refrigerated, for up to 2 days.

1 cup (250 mL) fresh blueberries

1 cup (250 mL) unsweetened almond milk (or homemade, page 23)

1 tbsp (15 mL) maple syrup

½ tsp (2 mL) latte spice mix

¼ cup (60 mL) chia seeds

1 small handful slivered almonds

CHOCOLATE, COCONUT, BLUEBERRY & RASPBERRY PARFAIT

This high-energy breakfast is well suited to be eaten about an hour before a workout. It's so delicious that it also makes a great dessert. Serves 1

 Transition   GF Gluten-Free

Prep Time: 5 minutes

½ cup (125 mL) chocolate ganache (page 40)

½ cup (125 mL) gluten-free rolled oats

½ cup (125 mL) raspberries

½ cup (125 mL) coconut cream (page 41)

2 tbsp (30 mL) unsweetened shredded coconut

1 tbsp (15 mL) cacao nibs

Spoon the chocolate ganache into a tall glass. Cover with the oats, then the raspberries and blueberries. Top with the coconut cream and shredded coconut. Garnish with cacao nibs and a few blueberries.

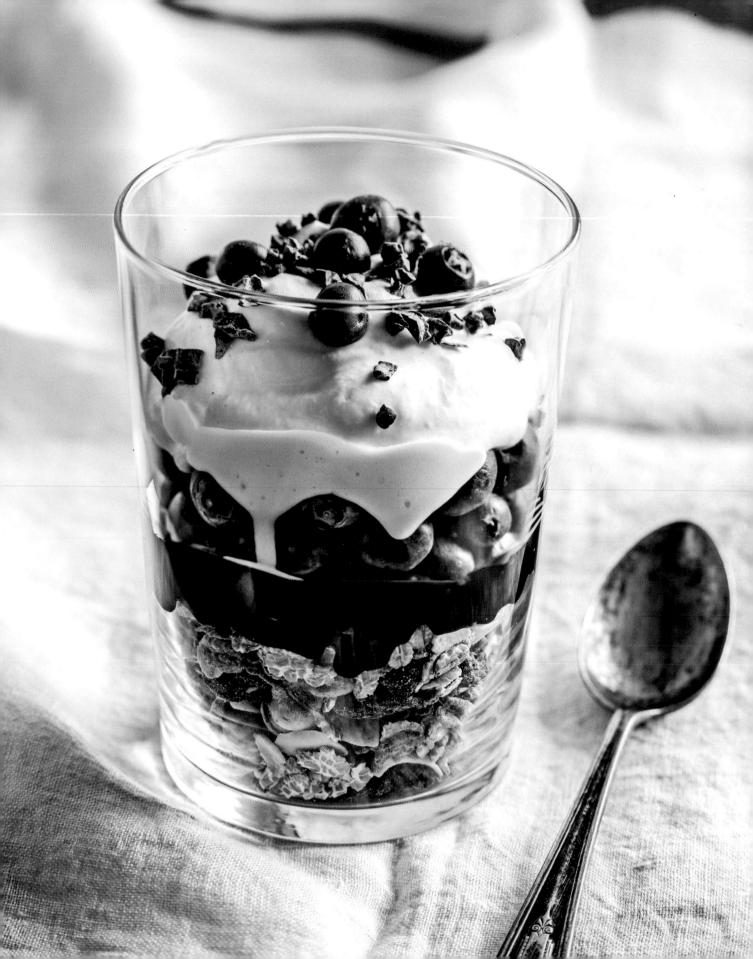

CHOCOLATE GANACHE

An ideal topping for those who are transitioning to plant-based clean eating. This recipe is wholesome yet decadent. Makes 1 cup (250 mL)

T Transition   **GF** Gluten-Free

Prep Time: 10 minutes • **Special Equipment:** blender

1 avocado, pitted and peeled

½ cup (125 mL) unsweetened almond milk (or homemade, page 23)

1 tbsp (15 mL) maple syrup or coconut nectar

1 tsp (5 mL) vegan dark chocolate chips

1 tbsp (15 mL) cacao powder

1 tbsp (15 mL) virgin coconut oil, warmed to melt

Combine avocado, almond milk, maple syrup, chocolate chips, and cacao powder in a blender. Blend until smooth. While the blender is running, add the coconut oil until emulsified.

• Keeps in an airtight container, refrigerated, for 2 to 3 days.

COCONUT CREAM

As versatile as it is delicious, this coconut cream goes well on just about anything, from French toast, to waffles, to soups, to desserts. As well, it's a good source of high-quality fat. Makes 1½ to 2 cups (375 to 500 mL)

 Gluten-Free

Prep Time: 5 minutes • **Special Equipment:** hand mixer or stand mixer

Chill a medium bowl.

Open the refrigerated can of coconut milk and discard any liquid.

Place the thick coconut cream in the chilled bowl. Beat until fluffy.

1 can (14 oz/400 mL) full-fat coconut milk, refrigerated for 6 to 12 hours

....

• Keeps in a sealed container, refrigerated, for up to 1 week.

Variations

Sweetened Coconut Cream: While whipping, add 1 tsp (5 mL) vanilla extract and 1 tsp (5 mL) maple syrup or coconut nectar.

Chocolate Coconut Cream: While whipping, add 1 tbsp (15 mL) cacao powder.

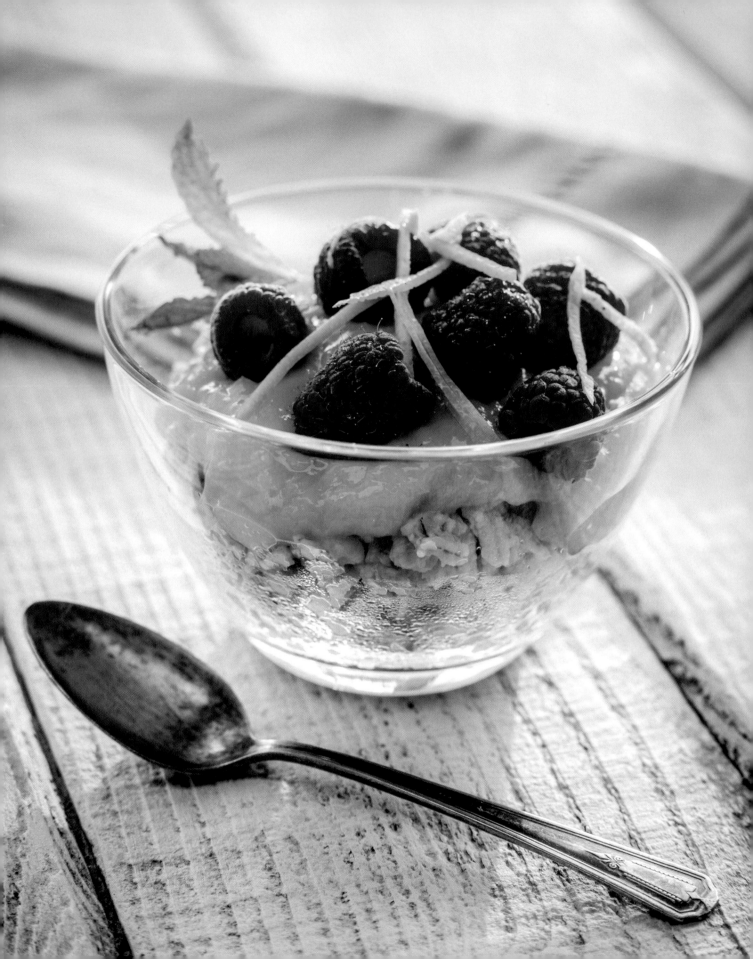

HOT OATMEAL WITH MANGO MOUSSE & RASPBERRIES

Citrusy and energizing, this breakfast digests easily and is bursting with antioxidants from the mango and raspberries. This hot oatmeal can be eaten as a breakfast side or as a stand-alone breakfast. It's ideal about an hour before a long bike ride or hike. Serves 1

 Gluten-Free

Prep Time: 10 minutes • **Special Equipment:** blender

For the mango mousse, combine all the ingredients except the coconut cream in a blender. Blend until thick and smooth.

Gently fold in the coconut cream (if using).

For the hot oatmeal, combine all the ingredients in a small saucepan. Cook over medium-high heat, stirring occasionally, until the water begins to evaporate, 5 to 7 minutes.

Place the hot oatmeal in a bowl and then generously spoon some of the mango mousse over the oatmeal.

Top with fresh raspberries.

. . . .

• Remaining mousse keeps in a sealed container, refrigerated, for up to 1 week.

¼ cup (60 mL) fresh raspberries

Mango Mousse

1 cup (250 mL) peeled and coarsely chopped mango

2 tbsp (30 mL) orange juice

2 tbsp (30 mL) maple syrup or coconut nectar

1 tsp (5 mL) agar powder

¼ cup (60 mL) coconut cream (page 41; optional)

Hot Oatmeal

1 cup (250 mL) gluten-free rolled oats

¾ cup (175 mL) unsweetened almond milk (or homemade, page 23)

1 tsp (5 mL) maple syrup or coconut nectar

¼ tsp (1 mL) pure vanilla extract

Pinch of sea salt

ON-THE-GO BREAKFAST

Simple yet filling. The sprouted bagel contains a big dose of protein, and the roasted garlic aïoli makes it taste delicious while boosting your immune system.
Serves 1

 Gluten-Free (Option)

Prep Time: 4 minutes

1 sprouted bagel (my favorite is Silver Hills Squirrelly bagel), sliced in half (or 2 slices sprouted bread)

1 tbsp (15 mL) edamame hummus (page 69)

1 tbsp (15 mL) roasted garlic aïoli (page 78)

2 slices tomato

½ ripe avocado, peeled and thinly sliced

1 small handful of sunflower or other sprouts

Toast the bagel. Spread the edamame hummus on the bottom half of the bagel and the aïoli on the top half.

Top the hummus with the tomatoes, avocado, and sprouts. Top with the top half of the bagel and slice the sandwich in half, if desired.

....

• Goes well with freshly squeezed orange juice.

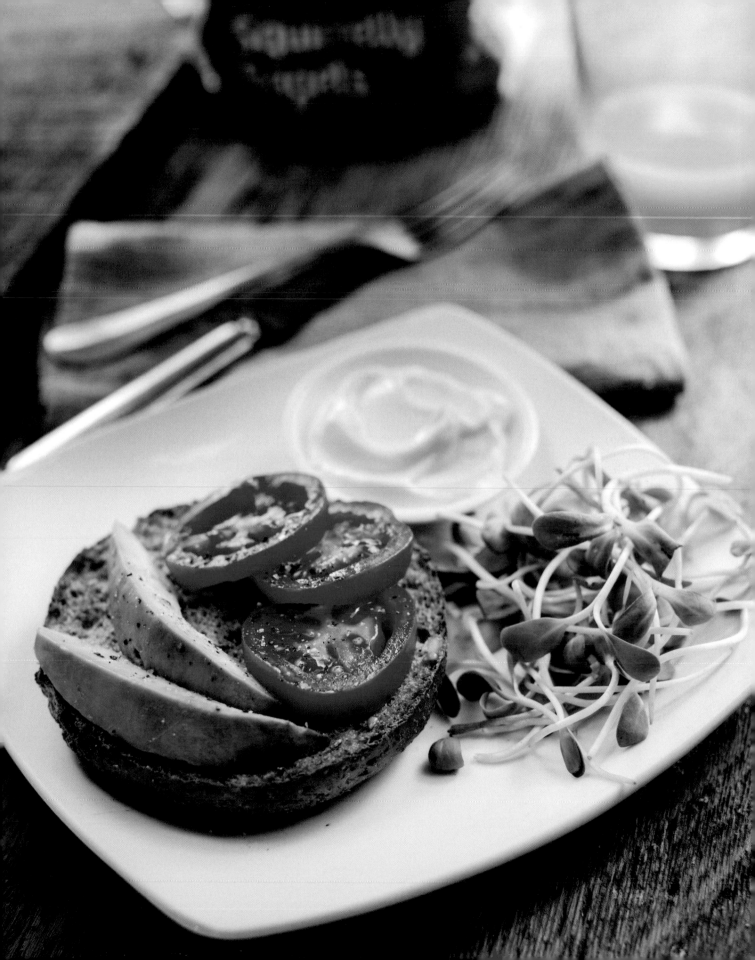

CRANBERRY ALMOND MUESLI CEREAL

This all-round delicious breakfast provides the staying power of almonds, chia, and oats. It will keep your blood sugar level stable so your energy level remains constant. Serves 6/Makes 6 cups (1.5 L)

 GF Gluten-Free

Prep Time: 5 minutes

4 cups (1 L) gluten-free rolled oats

½ cup (125 mL) dried cranberries

½ cup (125 mL) unsweetened shredded coconut

½ cup (125 mL) slivered almonds

½ cup (125 mL) sunflower seeds

¼ cup (60 mL) chia seeds

¼ cup (60 mL) agave nectar or maple syrup

1 tbsp (15 mL) cinnamon

1 tbsp (15 mL) virgin coconut oil, melted

¼ tsp (1 mL) sea salt

Preheat oven to 300°F (150°C).

Mix all the ingredients in a medium bowl and spread evenly on a large baking sheet. Bake the granola for 8 to 10 minutes or until it turns a darker brown. Let cool completely on the baking sheet.

Break apart before storing. Add 1 cup (250 mL) to a bowl and enjoy with your favorite nut milk.

....

• Keeps in an open container, refrigerated, for up to 3 weeks.

HOT APPLE PIE WAFFLE

Satisfying and delicious, these waffles are a Thrive Energy favorite.
Serves 1 or 2/Makes 4 large waffles

T Transition   **GF** Gluten-Free (Option)

Prep Time: 10 minutes • **Special Equipment:** waffle iron

For the waffle batter, in a medium bowl, combine the flour, baking powder, cinnamon, and salt. Mix together.

Add the almond milk and coconut oil; whisk until thick and smooth in texture.

Cook the waffles in a waffle iron according to the manufacturer's instructions.

Meanwhile, for the apple pie topping, combine all the ingredients in a small saucepan and cook over medium heat, stirring occasionally, until the apples have softened slightly, about 8 to 10 minutes. I prefer to not cook the topping too much, so the fresh taste and bite of the apples come through, but feel free to cook it down longer if you prefer.

Place the waffles on plates and add as much of the hot topping as you like. Drizzle with maple syrup and sprinkle with a little cinnamon. Add some coconut cream for extra flavor, EFA oils, and as a garnish.

• **Leftover topping keeps in a sealed container, refrigerated, for up to 1 week.**

Waffle Batter

1 cup (250 mL) whole wheat flour

¾ tsp (4 mL) baking powder

¼ tsp (1 mL) cinnamon

Pinch of sea salt

1 cup (250 mL) unsweetened almond milk (or homemade, page 23)

2 tbsp (30 mL) virgin coconut oil, melted

Hot Apple Pie Topping

2 medium apples, peeled, cored, and coarsely chopped

¼ cup (60 mL) maple syrup or coconut nectar

1 tbsp (15 mL) pure vanilla extract

1 tbsp (15 mL) virgin coconut oil

1 tsp (5 mL) nutmeg

3 tbsp (45 mL) maple syrup or coconut nectar, for garnish

1 tsp (5 mL) cinnamon, plus more for garnish

½ cup (125 mL) coconut cream, for garnish

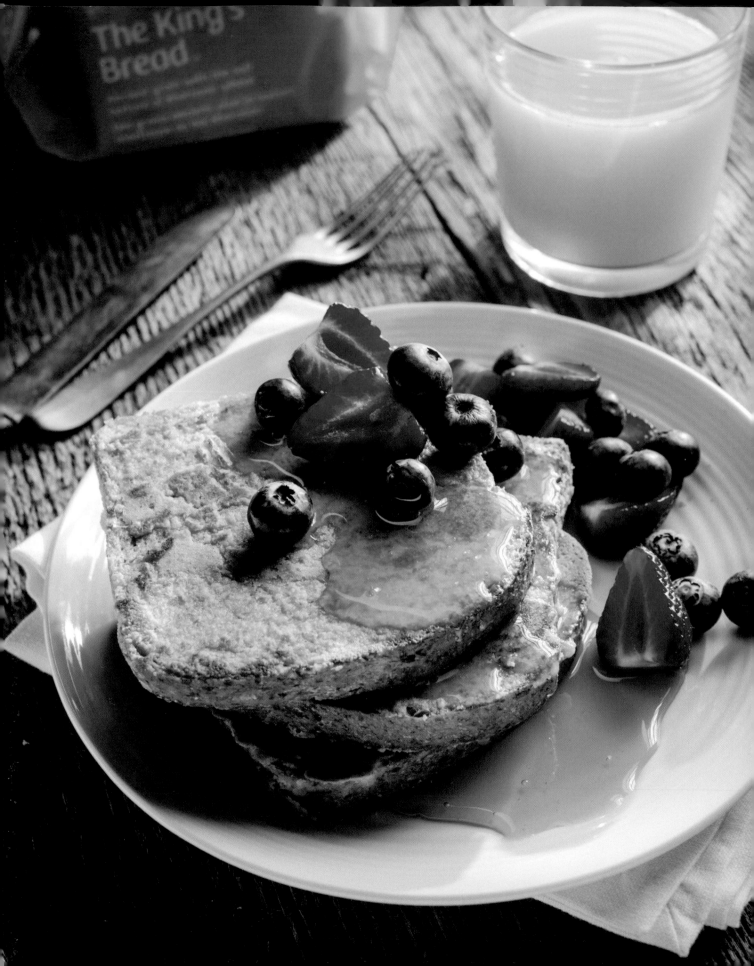

CASHEW BERRY FRENCH TOAST

Don't be scared off by the long list of ingredients. The flavor makes it all worthwhile. The deliciousness of this French toast has made it a Thrive Energy brunch favorite. Serves 2

GF Gluten-Free (Option)

Prep Time: 5 minutes • **Special Equipment:** blender, griddle

In a blender, combine the cashews, water, almond milk, vanilla, cinnamon, nutmeg, and salt. Blend until smooth. Transfer to a bowl.

Heat griddle to medium. Brush with coconut oil.

Dip both sides of the bread into the cashew mixture. Cook on each side until golden brown.

Top with coconut cream, fresh berries, and a drizzle of maple syrup.

½ cup (125 mL) raw cashews

1 cup (250 mL) water

1 cup (250 mL) unsweetened almond milk (or homemade, page 23)

1 tsp (5 mL) pure vanilla extract

⅛ tsp (0.5 mL) cinnamon

⅛ tsp (0.5 mL) nutmeg

Pinch of sea salt

2 tbsp (30 mL) virgin coconut oil

4 slices sprouted bread (my favorite is Silver Hills)

2 heaping tbsp (35 mL) coconut cream (page 41)

¼ cup (60 mL) fresh raspberries

¼ cup (60 mL) fresh blueberries

3 or 4 fresh strawberries, cut in half

2 tbsp (30 mL) maple syrup

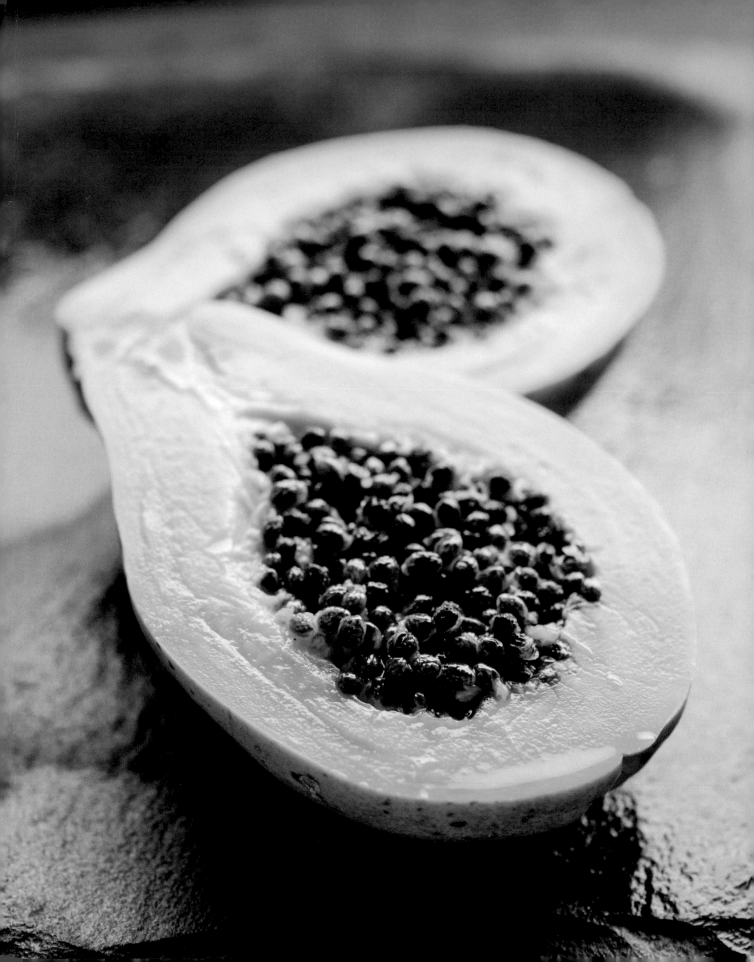

APPETIZERS,
SIDES,
SAUCES & DIPS

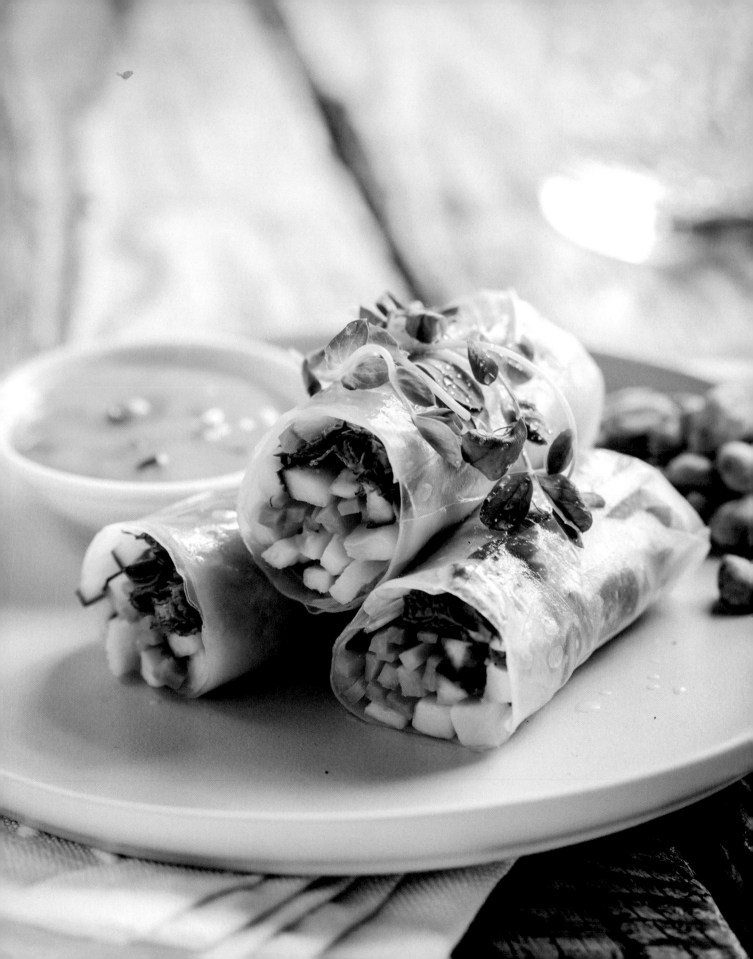

SUMMER ROLLS WITH MANGO LIME & MINT DIPPING SAUCE

Simple, light, refreshing, and packed with minerals, this take on spring rolls is a summer favorite. Serves 2 to 3/Makes 6 to 8 rolls

R Raw   **GF** Gluten-Free   **SND** Super Nutrient-Dense

Prep Time: 15 minutes
Special Equipment: mandoline with julienne blade or julienne peeler

Fill a large bowl with warm water and spread a kitchen towel on your work surface. Working with 1 rice paper wrapper at a time, soak wrapper in warm water just until pliable, about 30 seconds. Place it on the kitchen towel.

Divide the julienned fruits and vegetables and the kelp noodles evenly along the center of each wrapper, layering your ingredients as you go. Repeat with most of the cilantro, basil, and mint, reserving some for garnish.

Holding the end closest to you with both hands, fold it over the filling. Tuck it under the filling using your fingertips and gently pulling the wrapper taut. Fold in the sides, then tightly roll up the summer roll, squeezing the ingredients to get a tight roll. Place each roll as finished on a damp paper towel, and cover with another damp paper towel, to keep them from drying out.

Cut each roll in half diagonally and garnish with the remaining herbs. Serve immediately with mango, lime & mint dipping sauce.

6 to 8 rice paper wrappers (8 inches/20 cm or larger)

2 cups (500 mL) peeled and julienned mango

2 cups (500 mL) peeled, seeded, and julienned English cucumber

2 cups (500 mL) peeled and julienned carrots

2 cups (500 mL) peeled and julienned green papaya

2 cups (500 mL) kelp noodles

2 large handfuls of fresh cilantro with tender stems (cut off tougher bottom half of stems)

2 large handfuls of fresh Thai basil leaves

2 large handfuls of fresh mint leaves

½ cup (125 mL) of mango, lime & mint dipping sauce (page 74)

• If the rice paper tears while you're wrapping, just soak another wrapper and wrap it around the torn one.

GARDEN TAPAS PLATE

This snacking favorite is a mixture of Mediterranean-style ingredients and flavors, combined with nutrient-rich sprouts. Serves 2 to 3

GF Gluten-Free (Option)

Prep Time: 8 to 10 minutes

10 to 15 green or kalamata olives

10 to 12 slices paprika-marinated cucumbers (page 72)

¾ cup (175 mL) edamame hummus (page 69)

½ cup (125 mL) artichoke tapenade (page 68)

Small wedge of Cheddar cashew cheese (page 24)

8 cherry tomatoes, sliced in half

3 to 4 slices sprouted bread (I use Silver Hills Mack's Flax)

Small handful of sunflower sprouts, for garnish

Small handful of fresh sweet basil leaves, for garnish

Drizzle of extra-virgin olive oil or hemp oil

Place the olives, marinated cucumbers, hummus, and tapenade in their own separate ramekins. Arrange them on your serving plate along with the cheese and cherry tomatoes.

Slice each bread slice in half or quarters and arrange on the serving plate. Try to gain height by leaning the slices against a ramekin, for instance. Garnish the plate with sunflower sprouts and basil leaves.

Drizzle everything with some olive oil.

· ·

• **This dish should have a rustic look to it. Don't aim for perfection and symmetry here. Let the ingredients come together as a garden naturally would.**

RED LENTIL FALAFELS WITH ARTICHOKE TAPENADE

Satisfying and bursting with flavor, these falafels could also be served as a light meal.
Serves 3 to 4

PR Protein-Rich

Prep Time: 10 minutes

8 large endive leaves

½ cup (125 mL) artichoke tapenade (page 68)

2 cups (500 mL) quinoa tabbouleh salad (page 143)

Red Lentil Falafels

1 cup (250 mL) red lentils, rinsed

½ cup (125 mL) medium bulgur, rinsed twice

Sea salt

½ cup (125 mL) virgin olive oil or hemp oil, plus more for drizzling

1 medium onion, finely chopped

2 tbsp (30 mL) ground cumin

1 tbsp (15 mL) tomato paste

1 tbsp (15 mL) sweet red pepper paste

1 bunch green onions, finely chopped

1 large handful of fresh Italian parsley, chopped, plus more for garnish

4 or 5 fresh mint leaves, finely chopped

1 tsp (5 mL) red pepper flakes

Freshly ground black pepper

2 tbsp (30 mL) freshly squeezed lemon juice

For the falafels, in a medium saucepan, boil the lentils in 2 cups (500 mL) water until the water is almost all absorbed, about 15 minutes.

Turn off the burner, add the bulgur and sea salt to taste, and stir once. Cover and let sit until the bulgur has softened, about 10 minutes. Transfer to a medium bowl and let cool.

Heat the oil in a medium skillet over medium heat. Add the chopped onion and cook, stirring occasionally, until translucent, 3 to 4 minutes.

Stir in the cumin, tomato paste, and red pepper paste and cook, stirring, for another 2 minutes.

Add to the lentil mixture, which should be cool by now. Add the green onions, parsley, mint, and red pepper flakes. Season with black pepper to taste. Stir thoroughly. Form the mixture into small torpedo-shaped patties that will fit snugly inside the endive spears. Evenly spread about 1 tbsp (15 mL) of the artichoke tapenade inside each endive spear. Place 1 falafel patty in each spear. (You will not use all the falafels.) Drizzle with some lemon juice and additional olive oil. Garnish with chopped parsley and serve with a side of quinoa tabbouleh salad.

• **Remaining falafel mix keeps in a sealed container, refrigerated, for up to 4 days.**

edamame hummus

artichoke tapenade

jalapeño & lime guacamole

black bean, sweet corn & mango salsa

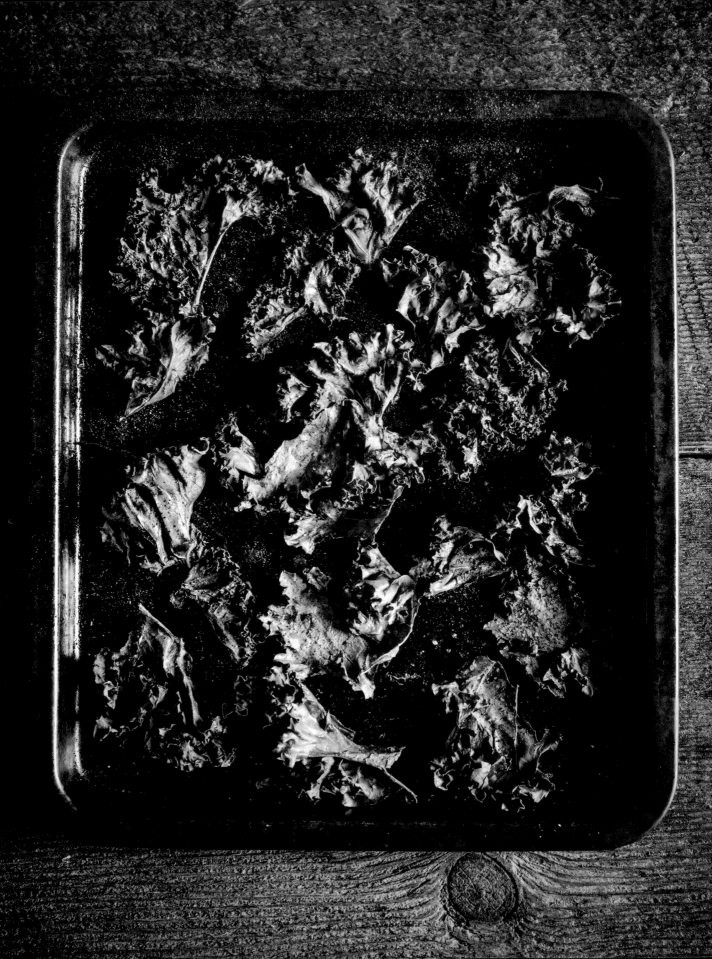

KALE CHIPS

An easy-to-make, simple snack that is flavor-packed and nutrient-dense. It's great for cutting cravings for calorie-laden snack foods. Serves 2

 GF Gluten-Free **SND** Super Nutrient-Dense

Prep Time: 5 minutes • **Special Equipment:** dehydrator (for raw version)

Preheat oven to 350°F (180°C).

Tear the kale leaves from the thick stems and tear the leaves into bite-size pieces. Wash kale, thoroughly dry with a salad spinner or kitchen towel, and transfer to a large bowl. Drizzle kale with olive oil and toss well or gently rub to thoroughly coat leaves with oil. Spread kale in a single layer on a baking sheet; some slight overlapping is okay. Sprinkle with fleur de sel or sea salt to taste.

Bake until the edges are brown but not burnt, 10 to 15 minutes. Alternatively, you can dehydrate the chips for 24+ hours.

1 to 2 bunches kale

¼ to ⅓ cup (60 to 75 mL) olive oil or avocado oil

Fleur de sel or sea salt

• Leftover kale keeps in an unsealed container at room temperature for up to 1 week.

TACOS WITH SALSA & GUACAMOLE

Fresh-tasting, satisfying, and bursting with nutrients, this twist on a traditional favorite has become a Thrive Energy staple. Serves 2 to 3/Makes 4 to 6 tacos

GF Gluten-Free   **T** Transition

Prep Time: 5 minutes

4 to 6 mini non-GMO corn taco shells

1½ cups (375 mL) jalapeño & lime guacamole (page 71)

1 cup (250 mL) cooked (or rinsed canned) black beans

1 cup (250 mL) sweet corn kernels

1½ cups (375 mL) cucumber, papaya & melon salsa (page 73)

1 cup (250 mL) cashew sour cream (page 68)

2 large handfuls of fresh cilantro leaves

4 to 6 lime wedges

Divide the guacamole among the taco shells, then layer with the black beans and sweet corn. Top with the salsa and a dollop of the sour cream, and finish with some fresh cilantro leaves. Squeeze a wedge of lime over each taco and serve immediately.

GRILLED ASIAN EGGPLANT

A simple yet flavorful way to add nutrition to sandwiches, burgers, salads, and rice bowls. Makes enough for 2 or 3 sandwiches or burgers

 GF Gluten-Free

Prep Time: 5 minutes • **Special Equipment:** barbecue or grill pan

1 large Asian eggplant, cut diagonally into ½-inch (1 cm) slices

¼ cup (60 mL) grapeseed oil

Sea salt and freshly ground black pepper

Preheat grill to high, if using.

Brush both sides of eggplant with oil. Season with salt and pepper to taste.

Grill eggplant, turning once, until grill marks can be seen, about 3 minute per side. (Alternatively, cook eggplant in a grill pan over medium-high heat.)

Let cool before serving.

GRILLED PORTOBELLO MUSHROOMS

These mushrooms can be used as a burger patty because of their meaty texture. Or cut them into strips to add flavor and texture to salads and sandwiches.
Makes enough for 2 to 4 sandwiches or burgers

GF Gluten-Free

Prep Time: 5 minutes • **Special Equipment:** barbecue or grill pan

6 to 8 medium portobello mushroom caps, stems removed

¼ cup (60 mL) grapeseed oil

Sea salt and freshly ground black pepper

Preheat grill to high, if using.

Brush both sides of mushroom caps with oil. Season with salt and pepper to taste.

Grill mushrooms, turning once, until grill marks can be seen, about 3 to 4 minutes per side. (Alternatively, cook mushrooms in a grill pan over medium-high heat.)

GRILLED ZUCCHINI

Grilled zucchini, full of flavor and nutrition, is an excellent addition to any sandwich or burger. Makes enough for 2 to 4 sandwiches or burgers

 Gluten-Free

Prep Time: 5 minutes • **Special Equipment:** mandoline, barbecue or grill pan

1 to 2 medium zucchini, cut lengthwise in ¼-inch (5 mm) thick slices on a mandoline

2 tbsp (30 mL) grapeseed oil

Sea salt and freshly ground black pepper

Preheat grill to high, if using.

In a medium bowl, toss the zucchini with oil and salt and pepper to taste.

Grill zucchini, turning once, until grill marks can be seen and zucchini is slightly limp but not overcooked, about 2 minutes per side. (Alternatively, cook zucchini in a grill pan over medium-high heat.)

Drain on paper towels and let cool. Cut in half, if desired, so they fit inside sandwiches.

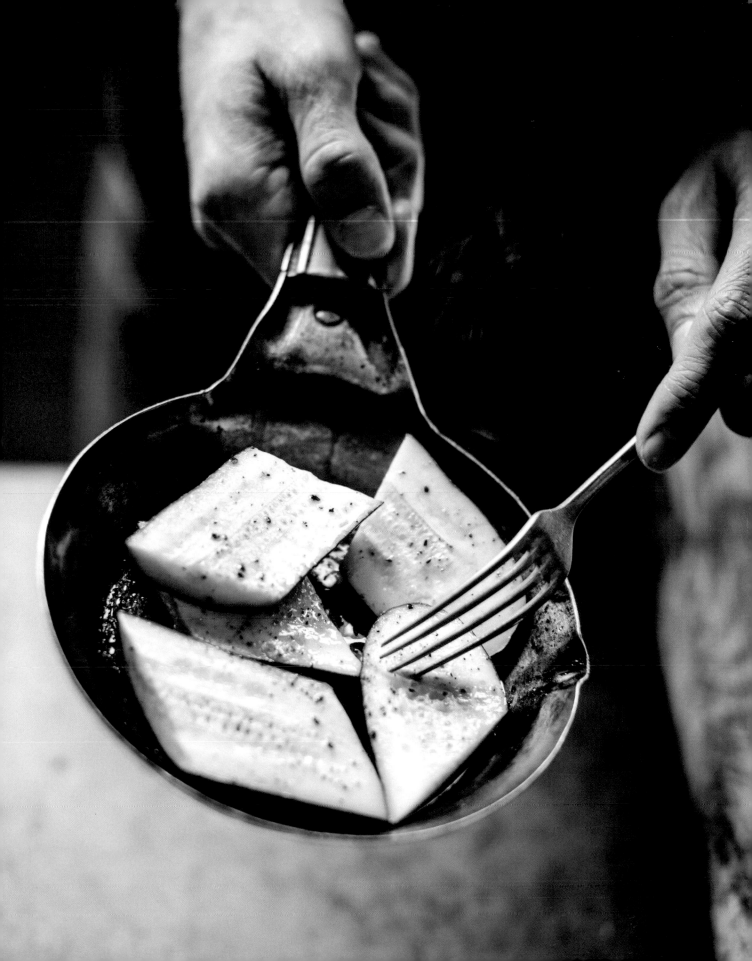

ROASTED GARLIC

A simple classic that adds flavor and immune-boosting properties to any meal.
Makes 2 cups (500 mL)

 Gluten-Free

Prep Time: 5 to 10 minutes

2 cups (500 mL) peeled garlic cloves

2 tbsp (30 mL) grapeseed oil

Pinch of sea salt and freshly ground black pepper

Preheat oven to 350°F (180°C).

In a small bowl, combine the garlic, oil, and salt and pepper. Toss to coat well.

Spread garlic on a medium baking sheet and bake until soft to the touch and golden brown, 20 to 25 minutes. Let cool to room temperature.

....

• Keeps in a sealed container, refrigerated, for up to 1 week.

BLACK BEAN VEGGIE BURGER PATTIES

Here's a classic protein-rich black bean burger staple. It's delicious paired with Cheddar Cashew Cheese (page 24). Makes 10 to 12 patties

GF Gluten-Free (Option)

Prep Time: 15 minutes • **Special Equipment:** blender

In a medium bowl, combine the black beans, oats, rice, nutritional yeast, and cheese. Mix thoroughly with your hands.

In a blender, combine the onion, cilantro, coriander, paprika, mustard, and tamari. Blend just until mixed.

Add the onion mixture to the bean mixture and mix well, adding salt. After mixing, adjust salt if necessary to taste. Add the bread crumbs and mix with your hands until the mixture is firm to the touch and no longer sticky. You will find that the bread crumbs and oats absorb the moisture and it will become harder to mix.

Form the mixture into ¾-inch (2 cm) thick patties.

Heat a skillet over medium heat. Add a little coconut oil. Fry patties until lightly brown, about 1 minute per side.

• Uncooked patties keep in a sealed container, refrigerated, for up to 5 days.

2 cups (500 mL) cooked (or rinsed canned) black beans

1 cup (250 mL) rolled oats

⅔ cup (150 mL) cooked whole-grain brown rice

⅓ cup (75 mL) nutritional yeast

¼ cup (60 mL) shredded Daiya or your favorite Cheddar-style cheese, dairy-free cheese, or Cheddar cashew cheese (page 24)

1 large cooking onion, peeled and grated (or chopped in blender)

1 large handful of fresh cilantro leaves, chopped

2 tbsp (30 mL) ground coriander

1 tbsp (15 mL) paprika

1 tbsp (15 mL) grainy mustard

2 tbsp (30 mL) tamari sauce

1 to 2 cups (250 to 500 mL) fresh bread crumbs made from sprouted bread (use Silver Hills Chia Chia bread for a gluten-free option)

Coconut oil

3 tbsp (45 mL) sea salt

RED LENTIL & CHICKPEA BURGER PATTIES

With its blast of nutrition and flavor, this burger is a favorite of those who are accustomed to being well satisfied at the end of a meal. This is an ideal burger if you are transitioning to plant-based clean eating. Makes 8 to 10 patties

T Transition   **GF** Gluten-Free (Option)   **PR** Protein-Rich

---

Prep Time: 15 minutes • **Special Equipment:** food processor

1 cup (250 mL) red lentils

3 cups (750 mL) cooked (or rinsed canned) chickpeas

1 large cooking onion, coarsely chopped

1 clove garlic, minced

½ tsp (2 mL) lemon juice

1 large sweet red pepper, finely chopped

1 handful of fresh cilantro leaves, chopped

1 large handful of fresh parsley, chopped

1½ cups (375 mL) cooked quinoa

1½ cups (375 mL) fresh bread crumbs made from Silver Hills or your favorite sprouted bread (use Silver Hills Rice Bread for a gluten-free option)

2 tbsp (30 mL) ground cumin

2 tbsp (30 mL) ground coriander

2 tbsp (30 mL) paprika

½ tsp (2 mL) freshly ground black pepper

3 tbsp (45 mL) sea salt

In a medium saucepan, boil the lentils in 2 cups (500 mL) of water until al dente, about 10 minutes. Drain, spread evenly on a baking sheet, and set aside to cool.

In a food processor, combine 1½ cups (375 mL) of the chickpeas, onion, garlic, and lemon juice. Process until smooth.

Transfer cooled lentils to a large bowl. Add the puréed chickpea mixture, remaining whole chickpeas, red pepper, cilantro, parsley, quinoa, bread crumbs, cumin, coriander, paprika, black pepper, and salt to taste. Mix well with your hands.

Form the mixture into ¾-inch (2 cm) thick patties.

In a skillet over medium-low heat, warm the patties for about 4 minutes per side.

. . . .

• **Uncooked patties keep in a sealed container, refrigerated, for up to 5 days.**

FALAFEL PATTIES

These are traditional-style falafels to help those who are transitioning to a cleaner plant-based way of eating. Serves 8/Makes 22 to 24 falafels

 T Transition   **GF** Gluten-Free (Option)   **PR** Protein-Rich

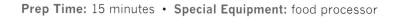

Prep Time: 15 minutes • **Special Equipment:** food processor

In a medium saucepan, boil the lentils in 2 cups (500 mL) of water until al dente, about 10 minutes. Drain, spread evenly on a baking sheet, and set aside to cool.

In a food processor, combine 1½ cups (375 mL) of the chickpeas, onion, garlic, and lemon juice. Process until smooth.

Transfer cooled lentils to a large bowl. Add the puréed chickpea mixture, remaining whole chickpeas, cilantro, parsley, bread crumbs, cumin, coriander, paprika, pepper, and salt to taste. Mix well with your hands.

Form the mixture into falafel patties 2 inches (5 cm) wide and ½ inch (1 cm) thick.

Heat a skillet over medium heat. Add a little coconut oil. Fry patties until lightly brown, about 3 minutes per side.

1 cup (250 mL) red lentils

3 cups (750 mL) cooked (or rinsed canned) chickpeas

1 large cooking onion, coarsely chopped

1 clove garlic, minced

2 tbsp (30 mL) lemon juice

1 handful of fresh cilantro leaves, chopped

1 large handful of fresh parsley, chopped

2 cups (500 mL) fresh bread crumbs made from sprouted bread (use Silver Hills Rice Bread for a gluten-free option)

2 tbsp (30 mL) ground cumin

2 tbsp (30 mL) ground coriander

2 tbsp (30 mL) paprika

½ tsp (2 mL) freshly ground black pepper

3 tbsp (45 mL) sea salt

Coconut oil, for frying

....

• Uncooked patties keep in an unsealed container, refrigerated, for up to 5 days.

ARTICHOKE TAPENADE

Packed with nutrient-dense artichoke and chlorophyll-rich basil, this is a favorite vegetable dip and burger spread. Makes 2 cups (500 mL)

GF Gluten-Free

Prep Time: 5 minutes • **Special Equipment:** food processor

½ cup (125 mL) pine nuts

2 cups (500 mL) drained canned artichoke hearts

2 or 3 fresh sweet basil leaves, thinly sliced

2 tbsp (30 mL) freshly squeezed lemon juice

2 tbsp (30 mL) avocado oil

1 tsp (5 mL) salt, or to taste

Pinch of freshly ground black pepper, or to taste

Combine all the ingredients in a food processor. Pulse to coarsely chop, then process until tapenade is almost smooth but still a little chunky.

• Keeps in a sealed container, refrigerated, for up to 5 days.

CASHEW SOUR CREAM

A delicious and simple alternative to traditional sour cream.
Makes ¾ cup (175 mL)

T Transition **R** Raw **GF** Gluten-Free

Prep Time: 3 minutes • **Special Equipment:** blender

1 cup (250 mL) raw cashews

2 tsp (10 mL) cider vinegar

1 tsp (5 mL) lemon juice

⅛ tsp (0.5 mL) sea salt

Place cashews in a medium bowl and cover with boiling water. Let stand for 30 minutes.

Drain cashews and transfer to a blender. Add vinegar, lemon juice, sea salt, and ¼ cup (60 mL) water. Blend, adding more water if needed to form a smooth texture.

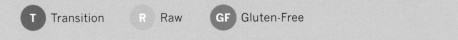

• Keeps in a sealed container, refrigerated, for up to 2 weeks.

EDAMAME HUMMUS

Rich in protein and phytochemicals, this hummus is an ideal dip for vegetables. It's also delicious as a burger topping to boost nutritional value. Makes 4 cups (1 L)

GF Gluten-Free   **PR** Protein-Rich

Prep Time: 6 minutes • **Special Equipment:** food processor

In a food processor, combine all the ingredients. Pulse to mix, then process until creamy smooth but thick enough to dip. Add a little water if it is too thick.

. . . .

• Keeps in a sealed container, refrigerated, for up to 1 week.

2 cups (500 mL) shelled edamame, thawed if frozen

1 cup (250 mL) cooked (or rinsed canned) chickpeas

½ avocado, peeled and chopped

3 small cloves garlic, finely chopped

¼ cup (60 mL) tahini

¼ cup (60 mL) freshly squeezed lemon juice

2 tbsp (30 mL) avocado oil

5 tsp (25 mL) sea salt, or to taste

½ tsp (2 mL) freshly ground black pepper, or to taste

½ cup (125 mL) water

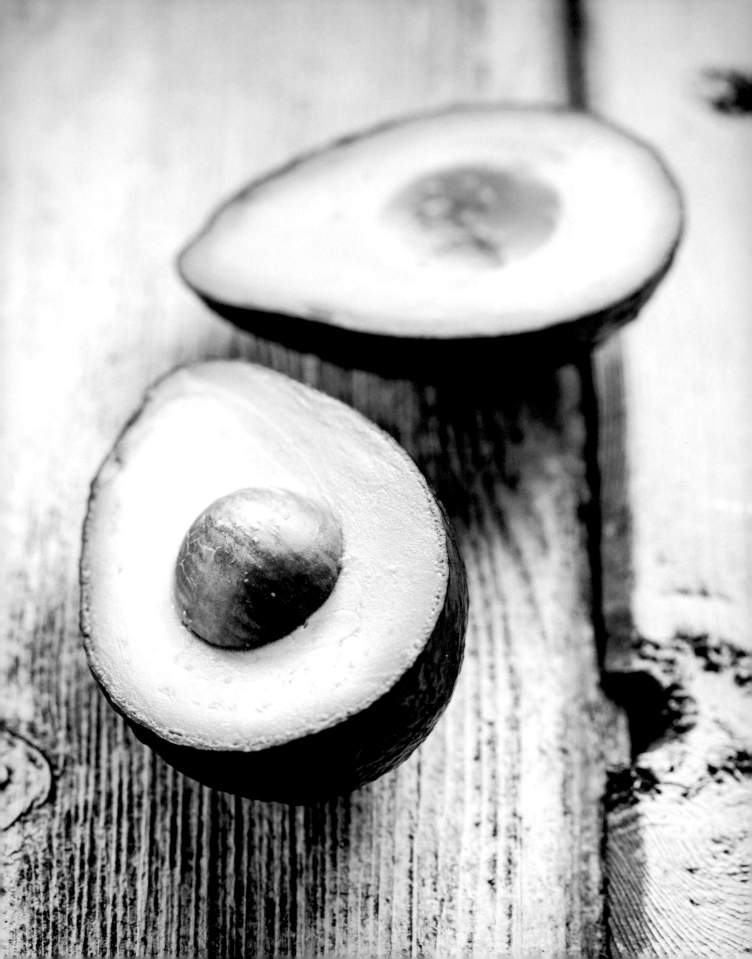

JALAPEÑO & LIME GUACAMOLE

Guacamole with a kick! This spread is ideal as a burger topping or a vegetable dip. Makes 3 cups (750 mL)

 Gluten-Free

Prep Time: 8 to 10 minutes

2 cups (500 mL) peeled and chopped ripe avocados

1 jalapeño pepper, seeded and minced

2 green onions, finely chopped

Large handful of fresh cilantro leaves, torn in pieces

4 or 5 fresh mint leaves, thinly sliced

2 to 3 tbsp (30 to 45 mL) freshly squeezed lime or lemon juice

1 tbsp (15 mL) hemp or avocado oil

Salt, coarse sea salt, or Himalayan pink salt, to taste

Freshly ground black pepper, to taste

In a large bowl, mash the avocados with a fork until smooth but still fairly chunky. Add all the remaining ingredients and gently stir together until well mixed.

. . . .

• Keeps in a sealed container, refrigerated, for up to 5 days.

PAPRIKA-MARINATED CUCUMBERS

An ideal side or topping for those who are transitioning to a cleaner diet, these cucumbers are full of flavor and have a nice touch of sweetness. **Makes 3 cups (750 mL) including marinade**

GF Gluten-Free

Prep Time: 5 minutes • **Special Equipment:** mandoline, blender

2 cups (500 mL) white vinegar

½ cup (125 mL) dark cane sugar

4 tsp (20 mL) paprika

1 medium cucumber, cut diagonally ⅛ to ¼ inch (3 to 5 mm) thick

In a blender, combine the white vinegar, cane sugar, and paprika and blend. The mixture should taste sweet yet sour. Depending on the type of white vinegar you use you might have to add more cane sugar if you feel it is not sweet enough.

Place the sliced cucumbers in a deep nonaluminum bowl and add the vinegar mixture. Cover and refrigerate. Use within 8 hours.

BLACK BEAN, SWEET CORN & MANGO SALSA

A twist on a southwestern classic, this salsa is bursting with protein and flavor. Try it with fresh vegetables or to top a salad. **Makes 3 cups (750 mL)**

R Raw   **GF** Gluten-Free   **PR** Protein-Rich

Prep Time: 6 to 8 minutes

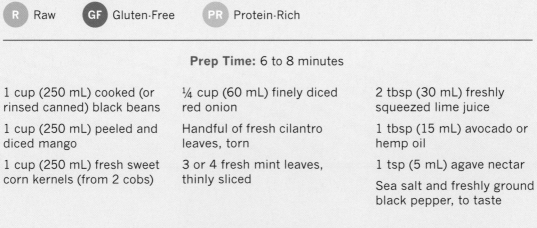

1 cup (250 mL) cooked (or rinsed canned) black beans

1 cup (250 mL) peeled and diced mango

1 cup (250 mL) fresh sweet corn kernels (from 2 cobs)

¼ cup (60 mL) finely diced red onion

Handful of fresh cilantro leaves, torn

3 or 4 fresh mint leaves, thinly sliced

2 tbsp (30 mL) freshly squeezed lime juice

1 tbsp (15 mL) avocado or hemp oil

1 tsp (5 mL) agave nectar

Sea salt and freshly ground black pepper, to taste

In a large bowl, combine all the ingredients. Toss well. Best served immediately.

• Leftovers keep in a sealed container, refrigerated, for up to 1 week.

CUCUMBER, PAPAYA & MELON SALSA

Rich in antioxidants, this fresh-tasting salsa can make just about anything taste great. Makes 3 cups (750 mL)

R Raw   **GF** Gluten-Free

Prep Time: 6 to 8 minutes

1 cup (250 mL) peeled and diced English cucumber

1 cup (250 mL) peeled and diced green papaya

1 cup (250 mL) diced cantaloupe

½ medium jalapeño pepper, seeded and minced

4 or 5 fresh mint leaves, thinly sliced

Handful of fresh cilantro leaves, torn

1 tbsp (15 mL) hemp or avocado oil

2 tbsp (30 mL) freshly squeezed lime juice

1 tsp (5 mL) agave nectar

Sea salt and freshly ground black pepper, to taste

In a large bowl, toss together all the ingredients. Best served immediately.

....

• Leftovers keep in a sealed container, refrigerated, for up to 1 week.

MANGO, LIME & MINT DIPPING SAUCE

Ideal as a dip and can also be used as a burger topping to give a kick of freshness.
Makes 1 cup (250 mL)

 Gluten-Free

Prep Time: 5 minutes • **Special Equipment:** blender

1 cup (250 mL) peeled and coarsely chopped mango

3 or 4 mint leaves, torn

Zest of ½ lime

1 tbsp (15 mL) freshly squeezed lime juice

1 tsp (5 mL) cane sugar

Combine all the ingredients in a blender. Blend on high until smooth and pourable.

• Keeps in a sealed container, refrigerated, for up to 1 week.

ROASTED GARLIC TAHINI SAUCE

This creamy, garlicky sauce can be used on anything savory that needs a flavor boost. Makes 1½ cups (375 mL)

 Gluten-Free

Prep Time: 4 minutes • **Special Equipment:** blender

1 cup (250 mL) roasted garlic (page 64)

1 cup (250 mL) water

¼ cup (60 mL) tahini

2 tbsp (30 mL) freshly squeezed lemon juice

2 tbsp (30 mL) cider vinegar

1½ tsp (7 mL) agave nectar

½ tsp (2 mL) sea salt

Pinch of freshly ground black pepper

In a blender, combine all the ingredients. Blend until smooth.

• Keeps in a sealed container, refrigerated, for up to 1 week.

BUFFALO SAUCE

The quintessential transitional sauce, this is a buttery-rich way to help make the switch from traditional foods to plant-based eating. Try it on burgers, in wraps, or as a dipping sauce for oven fries. Makes ½ cup (125 mL)

(T) Transition   (GF) Gluten-Free

Prep Time: 5 minutes

½ cup (125 mL) Frank's RedHot sauce or your favorite hot sauce

¼ cup (60 mL) Earth Balance Vegan Buttery Sticks or melted coconut butter (page 27)

Pinch of sea salt

In a medium bowl, whisk together all the ingredients.

• Keeps in a sealed container, refrigerated, for up to 1 week.

RANCH SAUCE

This nutrient-rich twist on the classic is great on burgers and sandwiches and makes a perfect dipping sauce. Makes just over 1 cup (250 mL)

(T) Transition   (GF) Gluten-Free

Prep Time: 6 minutes

1 cup (250 mL) Wildwood Zesty Garlic Aioli

1 green onion, minced

1 tbsp (15 mL) finely chopped fresh parsley

1½ tsp (7 mL) finely chopped fresh dill

½ tsp (2 mL) finely chopped capers

1½ tsp (7 mL) cider vinegar

1½ tsp (7 mL) freshly squeezed lemon juice

Sea salt and freshly ground black pepper, to taste

In a medium bowl, combine all the ingredients. Whisk until well blended.

• Keeps in a sealed container, refrigerated, for up to 1 week.

PAD THAI SAUCE

A functional twist to an old classic, this Thrive Energy favorite is as phytochemical packed as it is delicious. Makes 3 cups (750 mL)

 Gluten-Free

Prep Time: 5 minutes • **Special Equipment:** high-speed blender

1½ cups (375 mL) smooth peanut butter

½ cup (125 mL) raw cashew butter

6 tbsp (90 mL) chopped fresh ginger

2 tbsp (30 mL) chopped lemongrass

2 medium cloves garlic, chopped

2 tbsp (30 mL) tamari sauce

1 tbsp (15 mL) tamarind paste (optional)

1 cup (250 mL) water

¾ cup (175 mL) cider vinegar

½ cup (125 mL) freshly squeezed lime juice (from about 6 limes)

In a blender, combine all the ingredients. Blend on low to incorporate, then blend on high until sauce is smooth and creamy.

....

- You may need to add more water if your peanut butter is thick.
- Keeps in a sealed container, refrigerated, for up to 1 week.

REUBEN DRESSING

This flavorful dressing is terrific on a sandwich or burger—and of course on a salad. Makes 1 cup (250 mL)

 Transition   GF Gluten-Free

Prep Time: 5 minutes

In a medium bowl, combine all the ingredients. Whisk together until smooth and creamy.

....

• Keeps in a sealed container, refrigerated, for up to 1 week.

½ jar (16 oz/454 g) Wildwood Zesty Garlic Aioli

1 tbsp (15 mL) finely chopped chives

1½ tsp (7 mL) freshly squeezed lemon juice

1½ tsp (7 mL) organic ketchup

1 tsp (5 mL) vegan Worcestershire sauce

½ tsp (2 mL) prepared horseradish

1 tsp (5 mL) agave nectar

Pinch of freshly ground black pepper

CHIPOTLE LIME AÏOLI

Sweet, sour, savory, and spicy, this sauce spans the flavor spectrum. Plus, it supplies a solid nutritional kick. Great as a dip for raw vegetables or baked corn chips. Makes 2 cups (500 mL)

T Transition   **GF** Gluten-Free

Prep Time: 5 minutes

1 jar (16 oz/454 g) Wildwood Zesty Garlic Aioli

1 small handful of fresh cilantro leaves, finely chopped

1½ to 2¼ tsp (7 to 12 mL) finely chopped chipotle pepper in adobo sauce

1 tbsp (15 mL) freshly squeezed lime juice

1 tsp (5 mL) maple syrup or coconut nectar

1 tsp (5 mL) sea salt

Pinch of freshly ground black pepper

In a medium bowl, combine all the ingredients. Whisk together until smooth.

....

• Keeps in a sealed container, refrigerated, for up to 1 week.

ROASTED GARLIC AÏOLI

This aïoli provides the immune-boosting properties of garlic with intensified flavor. It goes well on burgers and sandwiches. Makes 2 cups (500 mL)

T Transition   **GF** Gluten-Free

Prep Time: 5 minutes • **Special Equipment:** high-speed blender

1 jar (16 oz/454 g) Wildwood Zesty Garlic Aioli

1 cup (250 mL) roasted garlic (page 64)

1 tbsp (15 mL) prepared horseradish

2 tbsp (30 mL) freshly squeezed lemon juice

1 tsp (5 mL) sea salt

1 tsp (5 mL) pepper

In a blender, combine half of the garlic aïoli with the remaining ingredients. Blend on high until creamy. Add 2 tbsp (30 mL) water if the aïoli is too thick to blend properly.

In a medium bowl, combine the remaining jarred aïoli with the blended aïoli. Stir until well mixed.

....

• Keeps in a sealed container, refrigerated, for up to 1 week.

WASABI AÏOLI

Immune-boosting with a kick. Makes a great dip, and goes especially well with baked sweet potatoes. Makes 1½ cups (375 mL)

T Transition   **GF** Gluten-Free

Prep Time: 5 minutes

1 jar (16 oz/454 g) Wildwood
Zesty Garlic Aioli

1 tsp (5 mL) wasabi paste or to taste

In a medium bowl, whisk together aïoli and wasabi paste, leaving no lumps of wasabi paste.

• Keeps in a sealed container, refrigerated, for up to 1 week.

YELLOW CURRY AÏOLI

A flavorful, nutrient-rich twist on classic curry aïoli that's great on burgers, as a light pizza sauce, or with rice. Makes 1½ cups (375 mL)

T Transition   **GF** Gluten-Free

Prep Time: 5 minutes

1 jar (16 oz/454 g) Wildwood
Zesty Garlic Aioli

1 tsp (5 mL) yellow curry paste

2 to 3 fresh or frozen curry
leaves, thinly sliced

Zest and juice of ½ lime

Sea salt and freshly ground
black pepper, to taste

In a medium bowl, combine all the ingredients. Whisk until smooth, leaving no chunks of curry paste.

• Keeps in a sealed container, refrigerated, for up to 1 week.

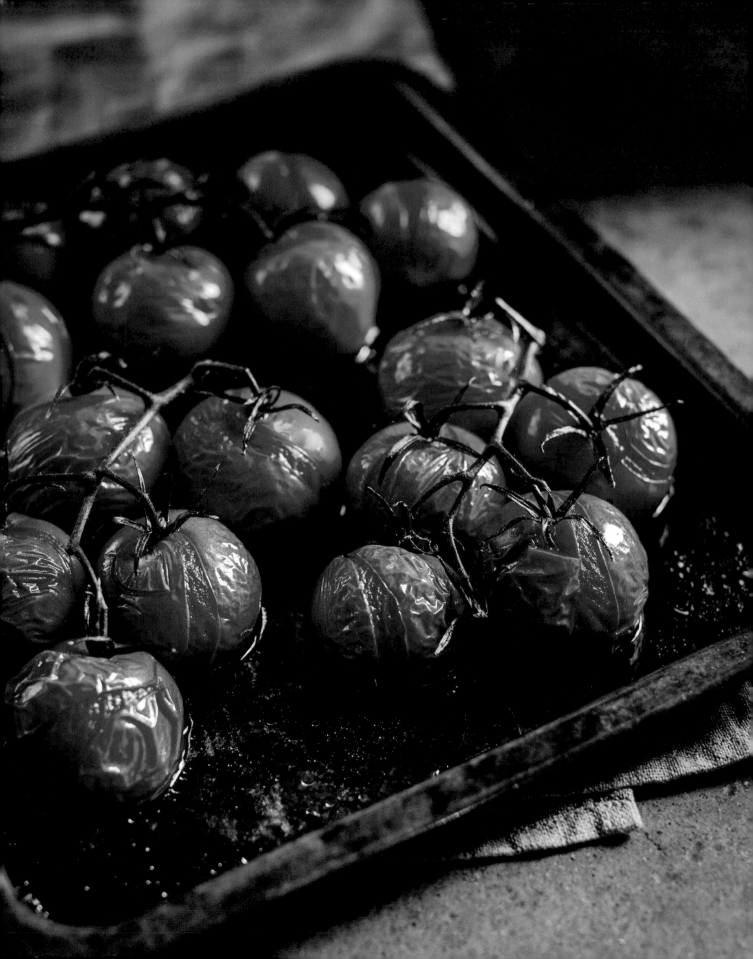

SANDWICHES, WRAPS & BURGERS

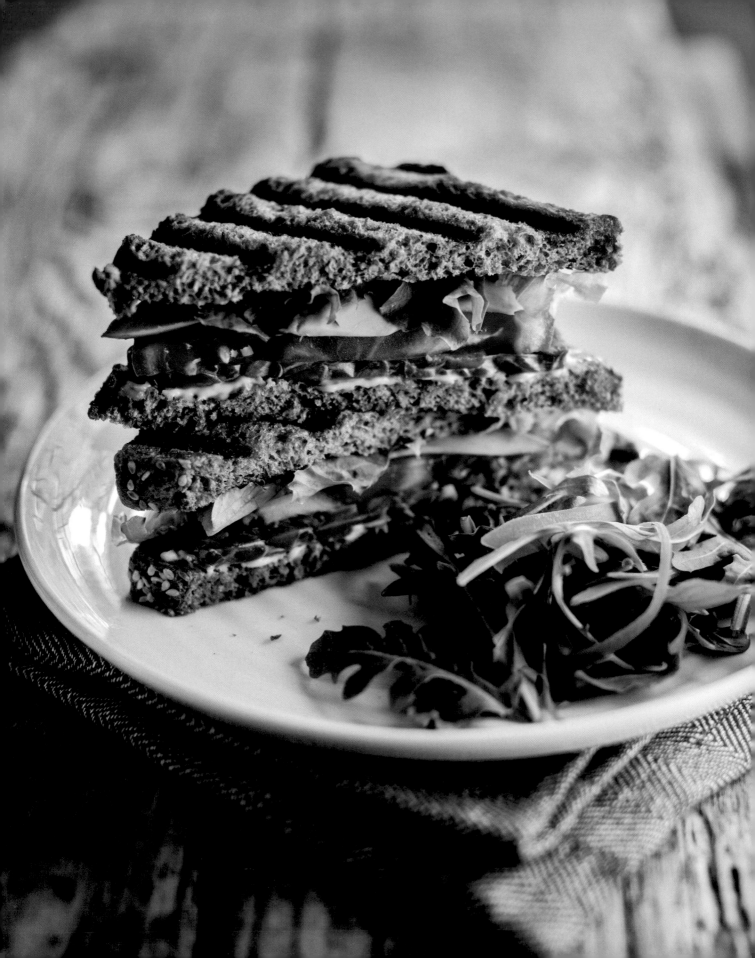

A.L.T. AVOCADO, LETTUCE & TOMATO SANDWICH

A Thrive Energy twist applied to a perennial favorite. This sandwich is as chock-full of nutrition as it is with flavor. Toasting the bread first in a panini press keeps the filling fresh and prevents the toast from becoming soggy. Makes 1 sandwich

T Transition   **GF** Gluten-Free (Option)

Prep Time: 5 minutes • **Special Equipment:** panini press or grill pan

Press the bread slices together and lightly spread some virgin coconut oil on the outsides. Cook in a panini press on medium-high heat until golden and lightly crisp, 3 to 4 minutes.

Pull the bread slices apart. Spread edamame hummus on the untoasted side of one slice and garlic aïoli on the untoasted side of the other slice. Arrange avocado, tomato, and tempeh over the hummus. Top with the spring mix and the top slice of bread. Cut the sandwich in half diagonally and serve with pickles.

. . . .

• You can use more roasted garlic aïoli if you choose. I do! I love it.
• I prefer smoky maple marinated tempeh from Turtle Island Foods.

2 thick slices sprouted bread (my favorite is Silver Hills)

Virgin coconut oil

1 tbsp (15 mL) edamame hummus (page 69)

1 tbsp (15 mL) roasted garlic aïoli (page 78)

¼ ripe avocado, peeled and thinly sliced

2 slices tomato

4 slices smoky maple tempeh, grilled on each side for 2 to 3 minutes

1 small handful of spring mix greens

2 medium dill pickles, quartered lengthwise, for garnish

REUBEN SANDWICH

A plant-based version of the classic sandwich, this flavorful Reuben is an ideal transition option for those who are in the process of cleaning up their diet. And it's even better with Cheddar Cashew Cheese (page 24). Makes 1 sandwich

 T Transition **GF** Gluten-Free (Option)

Prep Time: 6 to 8 minutes • **Special Equipment:** panini press or grill pan

2 thick slices sprouted bread
(my favorite is Silver Hills)

Virgin coconut oil

1 to 2 tbsp (15 to 30 mL)
Reuben dressing (page 77)

¼ cup (60 mL) shredded Daiya
or your favorite dairy-free
mozzarella-style cheese, or
Cheddar cashew cheese
(page 24)

¼ ripe avocado, peeled and
thinly sliced

5 or 6 slices tempeh, grilled on
each side for 2 to 3 minutes

3 large thin red onion rings
(optional)

⅓ cup (75 mL) sauerkraut

1 small handful of baby
spinach

2 large dill pickles, quartered
lengthwise, for garnish

Press the bread slices together and lightly spread some virgin coconut oil on the outsides. Cook in a panini press on medium-high heat until golden and lightly crisp, 3 to 4 minutes.

Pull the bread slices apart. Spread Reuben dressing on the untoasted side of one slice. Arrange the cheese on the untoasted side of the other slice, covering the entire surface. The heat of the toast will melt the cheese enough.

Arrange the avocado, tempeh, and onion rings (if using) over the Reuben dressing, then top with sauerkraut, baby spinach, and the top slice of bread. Cut the sandwich in half diagonally and serve with pickles.

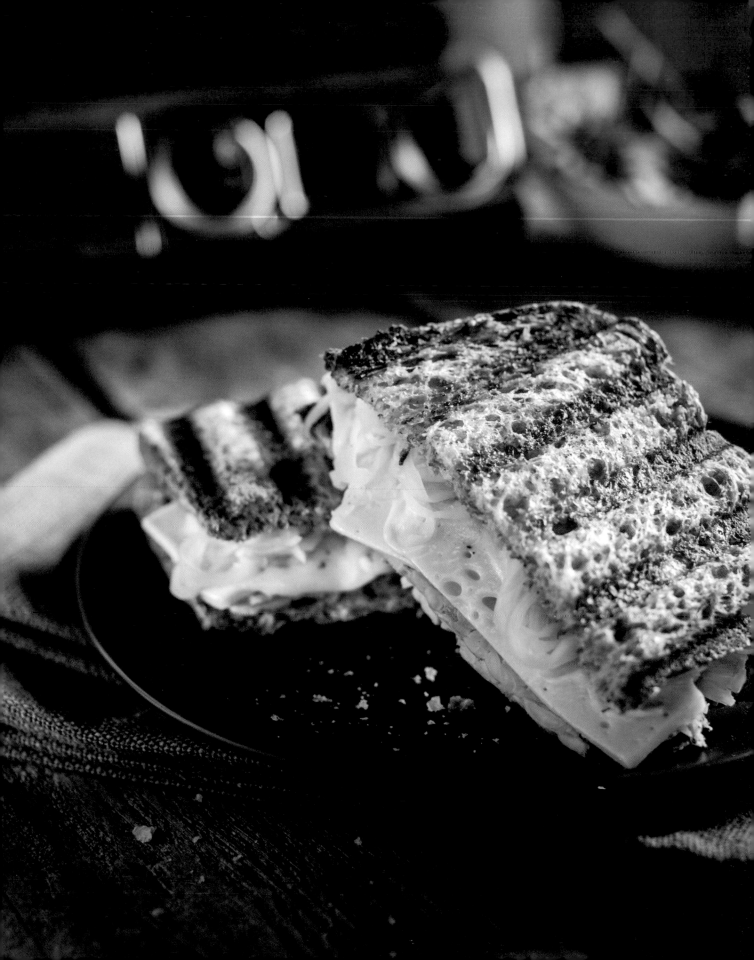

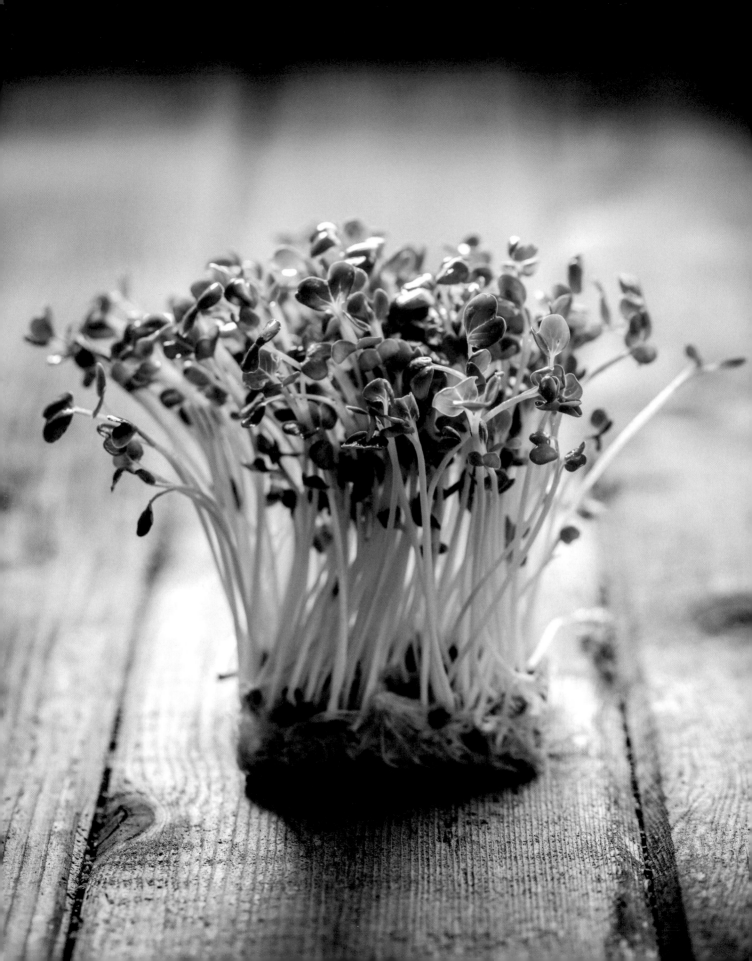

BIG GREEN SANDWICH

Fresh-tasting and stuffed with mineral-packed vegetables, this is a truly clean nutritious sandwich. Makes 1 sandwich

 Gluten-Free (Option)   Super Nutrient Dense

Prep Time: 5 minutes • **Special Equipment:** panini press or grill pan

Press the bread slices together and lightly spread some virgin coconut oil on the outsides. Cook in a panini press on medium-high heat until golden and lightly crisp, 3 to 4 minutes.

Pull the bread slices apart. Spread edamame hummus on the untoasted side of one slice and garlic aïoli on the untoasted side of the other slice. Arrange the zucchini, cucumbers, and avocado over the hummus. Top with the baby spinach, alfalfa sprouts, and the top slice of bread. Cut the sandwich in half diagonally and serve with pickles.

2 thick slices sprouted bread (my favorite is Silver Hills)

Virgin coconut oil

1 tbsp (15 mL) edamame hummus (page 69)

1 tbsp (15 mL) roasted garlic aïoli (page 78)

3 slices grilled zucchini (page 62)

4 or 5 slices paprika-marinated cucumbers (page 72)

½ ripe avocado, peeled and thinly sliced

1 small handful of baby spinach

1 small handful of alfalfa sprouts

2 medium dill pickles, quartered lengthwise, for garnish

GRILLED PORTOBELLO & TEMPEH SANDWICH

With a meaty texture and rich flavor, this sandwich is popular with those who are accustomed to more traditional sandwiches. Yet in true Thrive Energy fashion, it delivers a nutritional punch. **Makes 1 sandwich**

T Transition **GF** Gluten-Free (Option) **PR** Protein-Rich

Prep Time: 5 minutes • **Special Equipment:** panini press or grill pan

2 thick slices sprouted bread (my favorite is Silver Hills)

Virgin coconut oil

2 tbsp (30 mL) wasabi aïoli (page 79)

½ tsp (2 mL) Sriracha sauce, or to taste

2 to 3 grilled portobello mushroom caps (page 61)

4 slices tempeh, grilled on each side for 2 to 3 minutes

½ ripe avocado, peeled and thinly sliced

1 small handful of baby spinach

1 medium dill pickle, quartered lengthwise, for garnish

Press the bread slices together and lightly spread some virgin coconut oil on the outsides. Cook in a panini press on medium-high heat until golden and lightly crisp, 3 to 4 minutes.

Pull the bread slices apart. Spread wasabi aïoli on the untoasted side of each slice. Spread Sriracha sauce on one slice to desired heat. Top with mushroom caps, tempeh, avocado, baby spinach, and the top slice of bread. Cut the sandwich in half diagonally and serve with pickles.

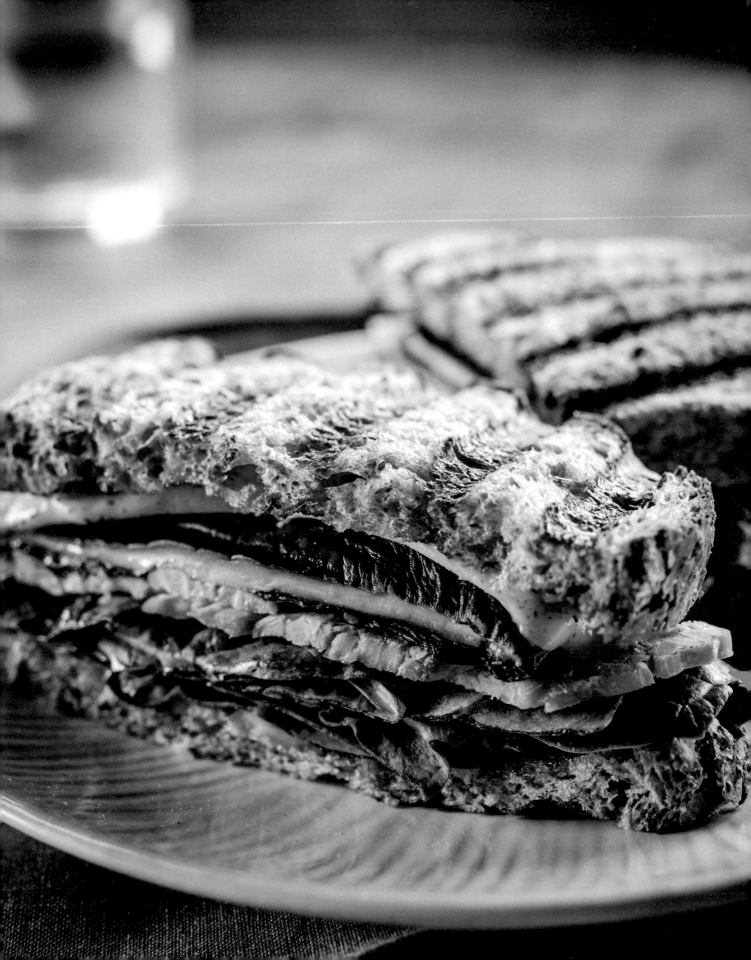

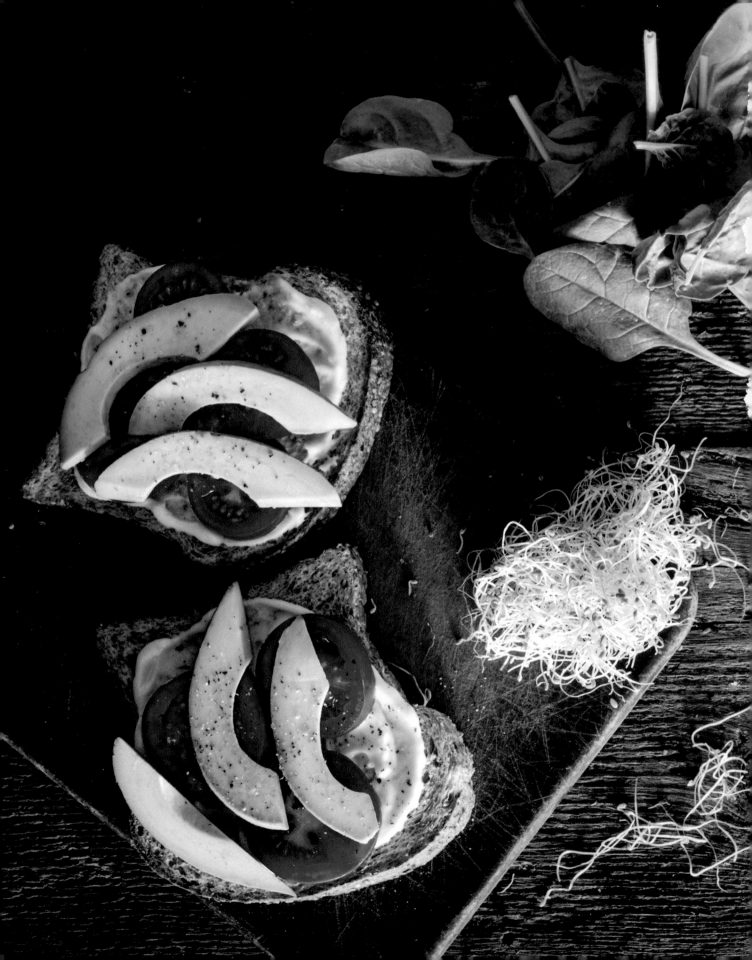

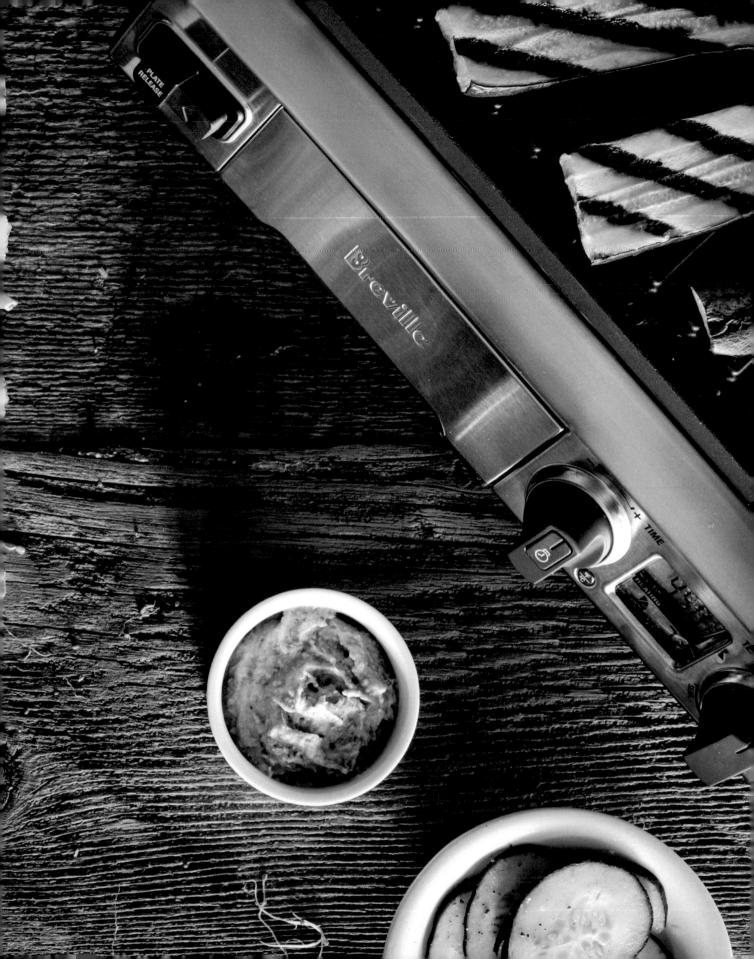

FALAFEL WRAP

With greens, sprouts, vegetables, falafels, and flavor-packed edamame hummus, this wrap is loaded with filling nutrition. Makes 1 wrap

 Gluten-Free (Option)   **SND** Super Nutrient-Dense

Prep Time: 8 to 9 minutes • **Special Equipment:** grill pan

1 Silver Hills or your favorite sprouted wrap (8 inches/20 cm or larger) or gluten-free teff wrap

2 tbsp (30 mL) edamame hummus (page 69)

2 tbsp (30 mL) roasted garlic tahini sauce (page 74)

2 large slices tomato

1 large dill pickle, quartered lengthwise

3 red onion rings

¼ cup (60 mL) diced English cucumber

1 small handful of fresh parsley leaves, torn

1 small handful of alfalfa sprouts

1 small handful of onion sprouts

1 handful of spring mix greens

1 lemon wedge

3 falafels (page 67), grilled for 4 minutes per side

Spread the hummus and tahini sauce over the middle of the wrap. Arrange the tomato, pickles, onion rings, cucumber, parsley, alfalfa sprouts, onion sprouts, and spring mix over the hummus and tahini, spreading them evenly.

Squeeze the lemon wedge over the greens. Top with the falafels. Roll up the wrap, tucking it in tightly with your fingers but not so tightly that you tear the wrap.

Heat a grill pan over medium heat. Place the wrap seam side down in the grill pan and cook for a few minutes to seal. Cut the wrap in half diagonally and serve.

BURRITO WRAP

Satisfying and loaded with fibrous nutrition, this southwestern-inspired burrito has become a go-to staple for those looking to load up on quality nutrition. It's a great option if you are transitioning from more traditional meals to clean, plant-based eating. **Makes 1 wrap**

T Transition   **GF** Gluten-Free (Option)   **PR** Protein-Rich

---

Prep Time: 8 to 10 minutes • **Special Equipment:** grill pan

⅓ cup (75 mL) cooked (or rinsed canned) black beans

¼ cup (60 mL) sweet corn kernels

1 large handful of fresh cilantro leaves, torn

½ large avocado, peeled and cut in medium dice

2 tbsp (30 mL) freshly squeezed lime juice

Sea salt and freshly ground black pepper

½ cup (125 mL) cooked wild rice

3 tbsp (45 mL) salsa (pages 72 and 73)

1 tsp (5 mL) ground cumin

1 tsp (5 mL) finely chopped chipotle pepper in adobo sauce

1 tbsp (15 mL) virgin coconut oil

½ black bean veggie burger patty (page 65), chopped

1 Silver Hills or your favorite sprouted wrap (8 inches/20 cm or larger) or gluten-free teff wrap

½ cup (125 mL) shredded Daiya or your favorite dairy-free Cheddar-style cheese, or Cheddar cashew cheese (page 24)

¼ cup (60 mL) diced fresh tomatoes

In a medium bowl, stir together the black beans, corn, cilantro, avocado, lime juice, and salt and pepper to taste. Set aside.

In a small bowl, stir together the rice, salsa, cumin, and chipotle. Set aside.

Heat coconut oil in a grill pan over medium heat. Add the chopped veggie burger and cook, stirring occasionally, until golden, 4 to 5 minutes.

Spread the rice mixture evenly down the middle of the wrap. Top with the grilled veggie burger. Top with the black bean mixture, avoiding any liquid in the bowl. Sprinkle evenly with the cheese and tomatoes. Roll up the wrap tightly but not so tightly that you tear the wrap.

Heat the grill pan over medium heat. Place the wrap seam side down in the grill pan and cook for a few minutes to seal. Cut the wrap in half diagonally and serve.

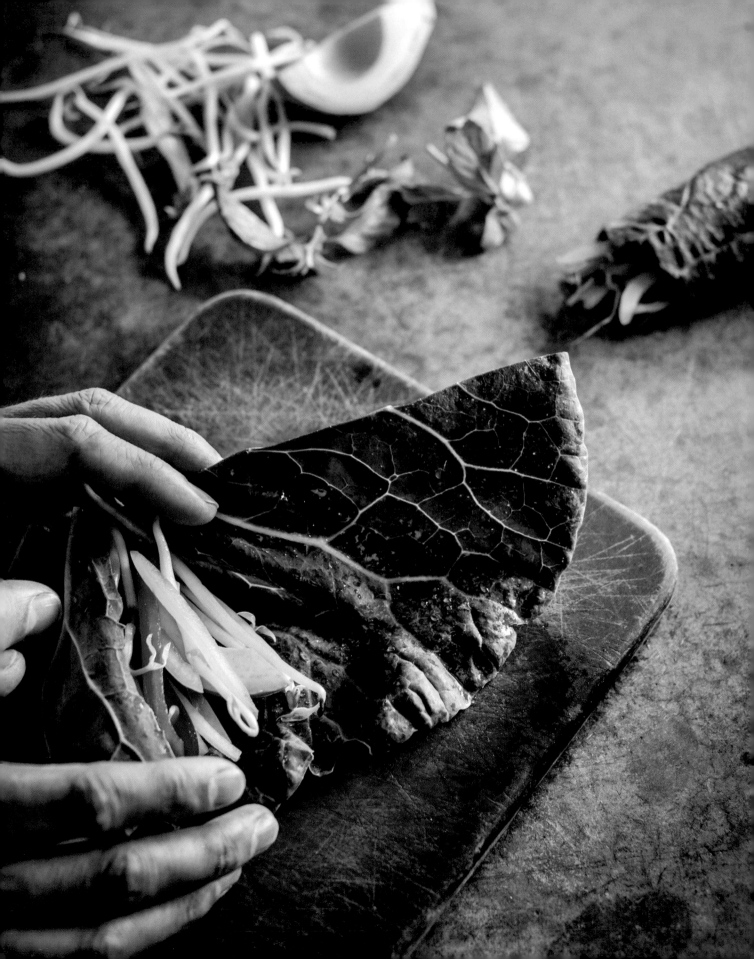

THAI WRAP

This wrap delivers an inspired but traditional Thai flavor. Rich in minerals and chlorophyll, it's jam-packed with nutrients that reduce inflammation.

Makes 1 wrap

R Raw   **GF** Gluten-Free (Option)   **SND** Super Nutrient-Dense

---

Prep Time: 6 to 8 minutes • **Special Equipment:** grill pan

Spread the sweet chili sauce and Sriracha sauce over the middle of the wrap. Arrange the avocado slices down the middle of the wrap. Top with the bean sprouts, basil, mint, and cilantro. Arrange the tempeh slices diagonally down the middle about an inch (2.5 cm) apart.

In a medium bowl, combine the Asian vegetable mix, lime juice, and garlic aïoli (if using). Toss well. Place the veg mix evenly down the middle of the wrap. Roll up the wrap, tucking it snugly but not too tightly with your fingers.

Heat a grill pan over medium heat. Place the wrap seam side down in the grill pan and cook for a few minutes to seal. Cut the wrap in half diagonally and serve.

. . . .

• **I prefer sesame garlic marinated tempeh by Turtle Island Foods.**

1 Silver Hills or your favorite sprouted wrap (8 inches/20 cm or larger) or collard green leaf

2 tbsp (30 mL) sweet chili sauce

1 tsp (5 mL) Sriracha sauce, or to taste

¼ ripe avocado, peeled and thinly sliced

1 small handful of bean sprouts

4 or 5 fresh Thai basil leaves, torn

4 or 5 fresh mint leaves, torn

8 to 10 fresh cilantro leaves, torn

3 slices tempeh, grilled on each side for 2 to 3 minutes

1 cup (250 mL) Asian julienned vegetable mix (page 128)

1 tbsp (15 mL) freshly squeezed lime juice

1 tbsp (15 mL) Wildwood Zesty Garlic Aioli (optional)

BLACK BEAN CHIPOTLE QUESADILLA

A southwestern classic updated with functional nutrition. Makes 1 quesadilla

GF Gluten-Free (Option)

Prep Time: 8 to 10 minutes

2 Silver Hills or your favorite sprouted tortillas (8 inches/20 cm or larger) or gluten-free teff wraps

2 tbsp (30 mL) chipotle lime aïoli (page 78)

3 tbsp (45 mL) salsa

3 slices tempeh, grilled on each side for 2 to 3 minutes (optional)

½ cup (125 mL) shredded Daiya or your favorite dairy-free Cheddar-style cheese, or Cheddar cashew cheese (page 24)

½ large ripe avocado, peeled and cut in medium dice

¼ cup (60 mL) diced fresh tomatoes

¼ cup (60 mL) sweet corn kernels

8 to 10 thin slices of jalapeño pepper, seeded

1 large handful of fresh cilantro leaves, torn

½ lime

Sea salt and freshly ground black pepper

Preheat oven to 350°F (180°C).

Place 1 tortilla on a medium baking sheet. Spread the chipotle lime aïoli evenly over the tortilla. Top evenly with the salsa.

Chop the tempeh (if using) and evenly sprinkle the pieces over the tortilla. Top evenly with the cheese, avocado, tomatoes, corn, jalapeño, and cilantro. Squeeze some lime juice over the filling. Season with salt and pepper to taste. Cover with the remaining wrap, pressing firmly to smooth out the surface.

Bake until golden, about 10 minutes. Cut into quarters and serve.

BUFFALO BURGER

This satisfying Thrive Energy go-to burger is delicious. Load it up with greens to pack in the nutrition. Makes 1 burger

 Transition　　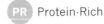 Gluten-Free (Option)　　PR Protein-Rich

---

Prep Time: 5 minutes · **Special Equipment:** grill pan

Preheat oven to 350°F (180°C).

Heat the coconut oil in a grill pan over medium heat. Cook the veggie patty for 4 to 6 minutes per side or until golden brown.

Cut the bun in half and put cheese on the top half; bake for 3 to 4 minutes until cheese is melted and bun is lightly golden. Spread the bottom half with the ranch sauce. Drizzle with the buffalo sauce. Top with the veggie burger, zucchini, red pepper, arugula, and the top half of the bun.

1 tbsp (15 mL) virgin coconut oil

1 black bean veggie burger patty (page 65)

1 sprouted ancient grain burger bun (my favorite is Silver Hills)

¼ cup (60 mL) pepperjack-style Daiya or your favorite dairy-free Cheddar-style cheese, or Cheddar cashew cheese (page 24)

2 tbsp (30 mL) ranch sauce (page 75)

1 tbsp (15 mL) buffalo sauce (page 75)

3 slices grilled zucchini (page 62)

½ roasted red pepper, cut in thin strips

1 small handful of baby arugula

AVOCADO, BLACK BEAN & CHIPOTLE BURGER

This popular Thrive Energy burger packs an explosion of flavor while retaining its nutritional functionality. Ideal for those who are transitioning to clean, plant-based eating. Serve with baked root vegetable chips, if desired. **Makes 1 burger**

T Transition   **GF** Gluten-Free (Option)   **PR** Protein-Rich

Prep Time: 5 minutes • **Special Equipment:** grill pan

Preheat oven to 350°F (180°C).

Heat the coconut oil in a grill pan over medium heat. Cook the veggie patty for 4 to 6 minutes per side or until golden brown.

Meanwhile, cut the bun in half and place cut sides up on a baking sheet. Sprinkle the cheese over the top half. Bake until the cheese begins to melt, 4 to 5 minutes. Then spread the chipotle lime aïoli on the bottom half.

Place the patty on the bottom half of the bun. Top with the tomato, avocado, lettuce, and the top half of the bun.

1 tbsp (15 mL) virgin coconut oil

1 black bean veggie burger patty (page 65)

1 sprouted ancient grain burger bun (my favorite is Silver Hills)

2 tbsp (30 mL) chipotle lime aïoli (page 78)

¼ cup (60 mL) Daiya or your favorite dairy-free Cheddar-style cheese, or Cheddar cashew cheese (page 24)

2 slices tomato

½ ripe avocado, peeled and thinly sliced

1 large romaine lettuce leaf

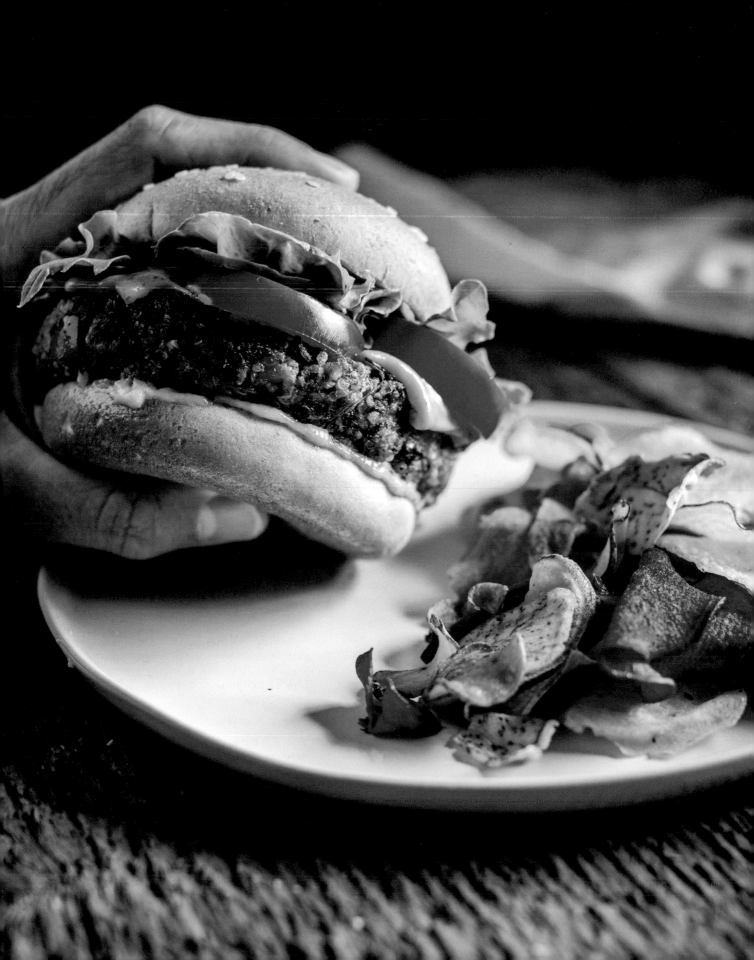

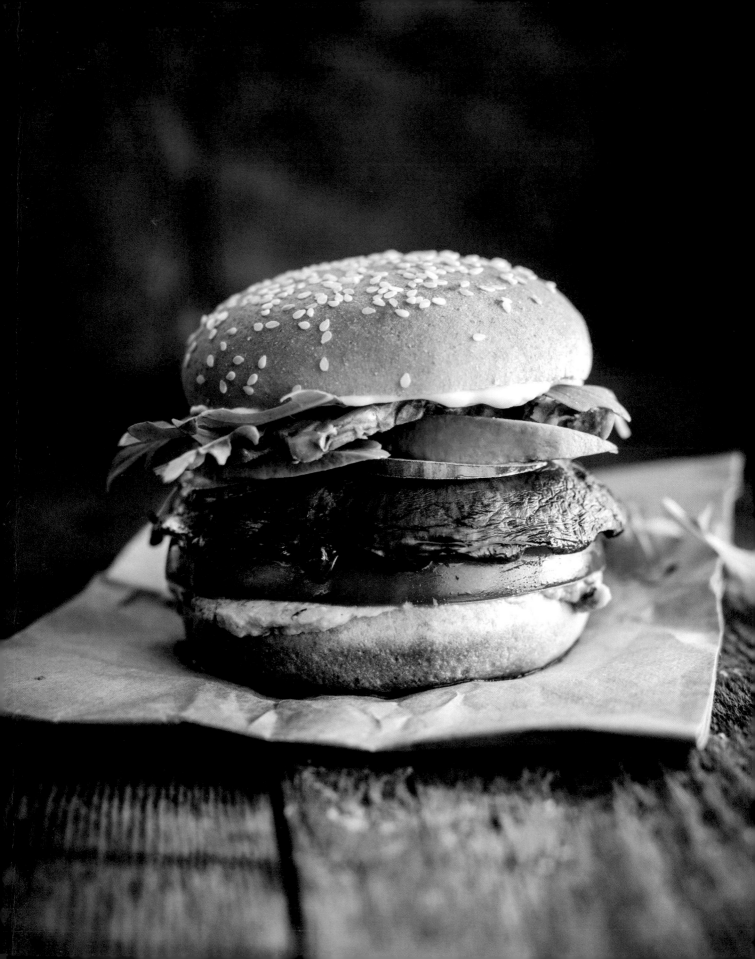

PORTOBELLO BURGER

A simple, mineral-rich burger with a meaty texture and earthy warmth.
Makes 1 burger

 Gluten-Free (Option)

Prep Time: 5 to 6 minutes • **Special Equipment:** grill pan, mandoline

Cut the bun in half. Evenly spread the bottom half with the edamame hummus and Sriracha sauce and the top half with the wasabi aïoli.

Top the hummus with the baby spinach, then layer with the mushroom cap, avocado, and fennel, and the top half of the bun.

1 sprouted ancient grain burger bun (my favorite is Silver Hills)

1 tbsp (15 mL) edamame hummus (page 69)

1½ tsp (7 mL) Sriracha hot sauce or to taste

1 tbsp (15 mL) wasabi aïoli (page 79)

1 small handful of baby spinach

1 large or two small grilled portobello mushroom caps (page 61)

¼ ripe avocado, peeled and thinly sliced

3 paper-thin slices fennel

RED LENTIL & CHICKPEA BURGER WITH YELLOW CURRY AÏOLI

Nutrient-packed and delicious, this burger is loaded with hearty goodness to keep you satisfied for hours without getting drowsy. A great burger for lunch that will take you through the afternoon. Makes 1 burger

GF Gluten-Free (Option)   **PR** Protein-Rich

Prep Time: 5 minutes • **Special Equipment:** grill pan

1 sprouted ancient grain burger bun or seedy kaiser roll

2 tbsp (30 mL) artichoke tapenade (page 68)

1 tbsp (15 mL) yellow curry aïoli (page 79)

1 red lentil & chickpea burger (page 66)

½ avocado, sliced thinly

3 slices grilled Asian eggplant (page 61; optional)

¼ sweet red pepper, thinly sliced

3 or 4 lettuce leaves

Heat the coconut oil in a grill pan over medium heat. Cook the chickpea patty for 4 to 6 minutes per side or until golden brown.

Cut the bun in half and evenly spread the bottom half with the artichoke tapenade and the bottom half with the yellow curry aïoli. Top with the red lentil & chickpea burger, avocado, Asian eggplant (if using), red pepper, lettuce, and the top half of the bun.

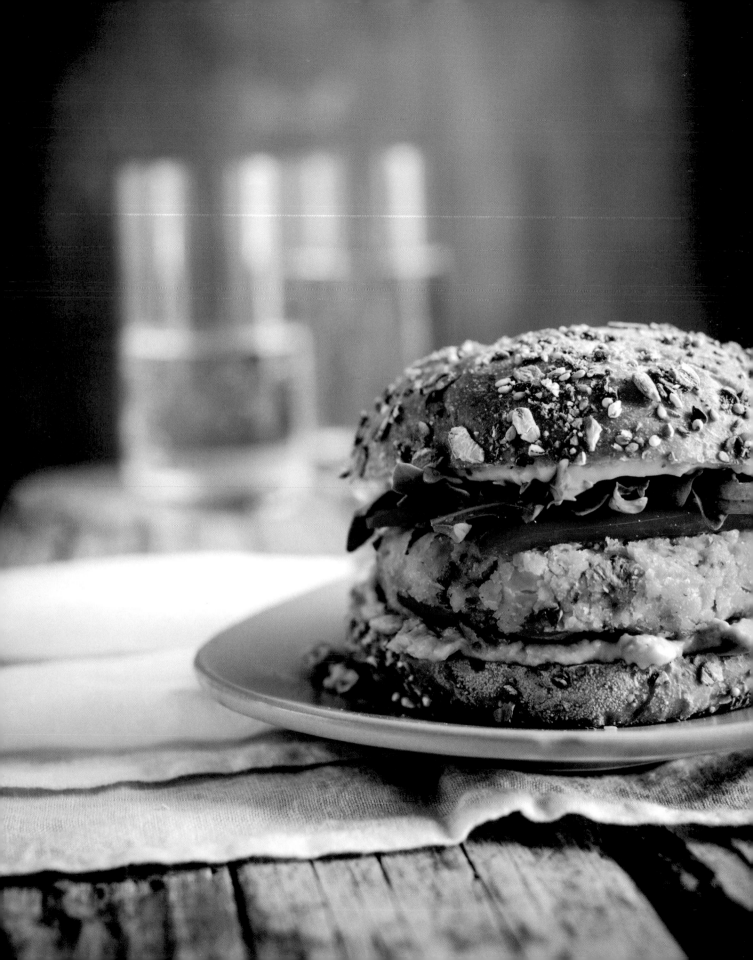

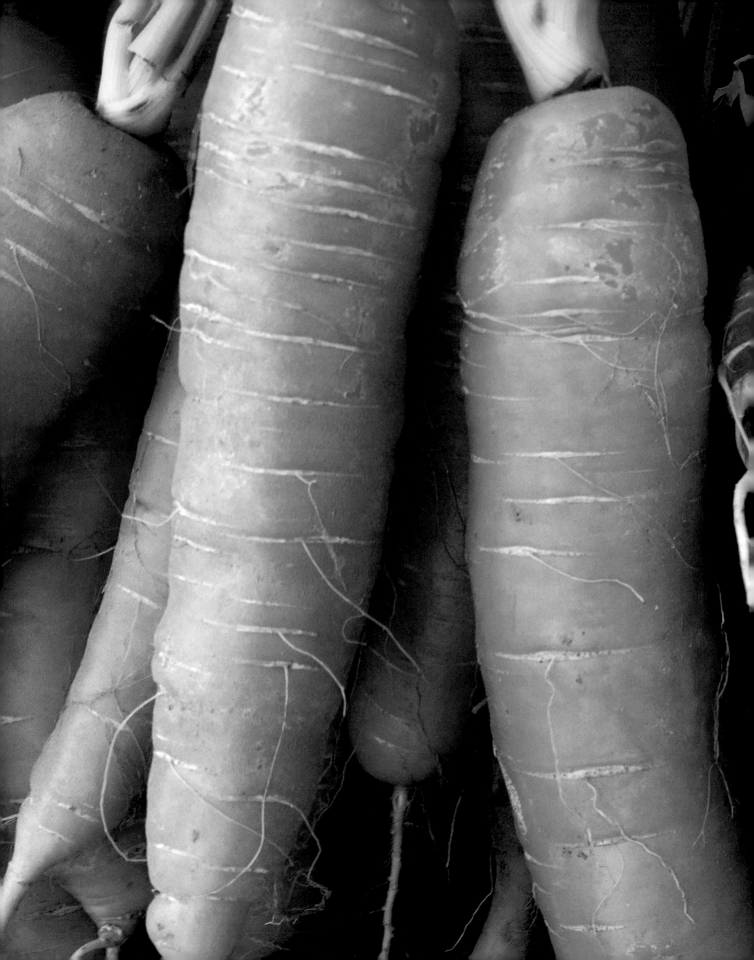

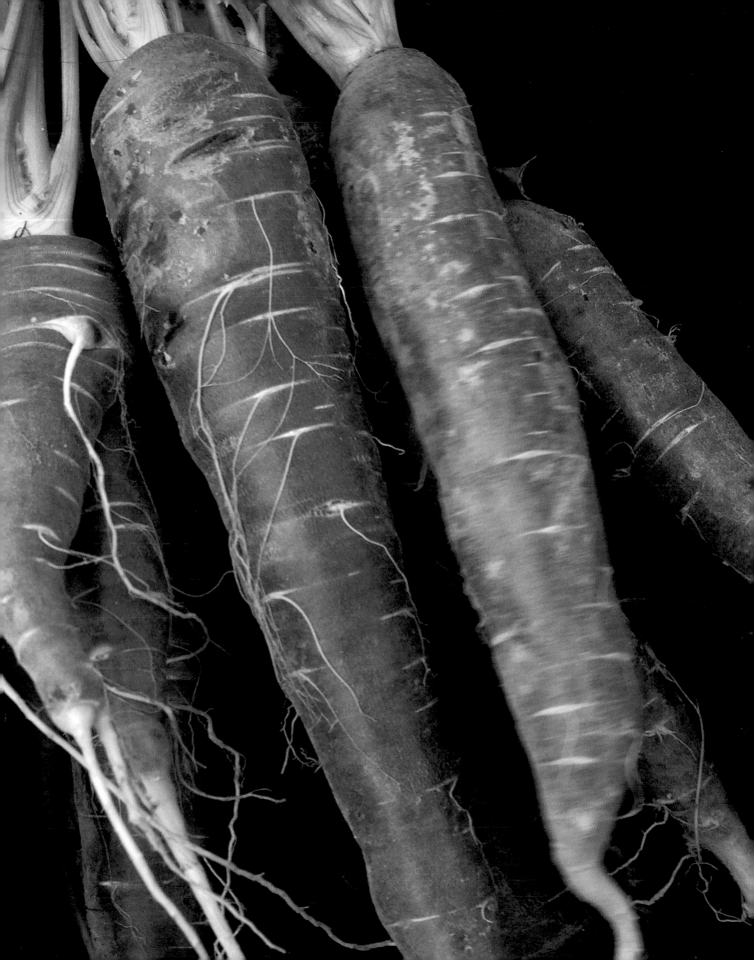

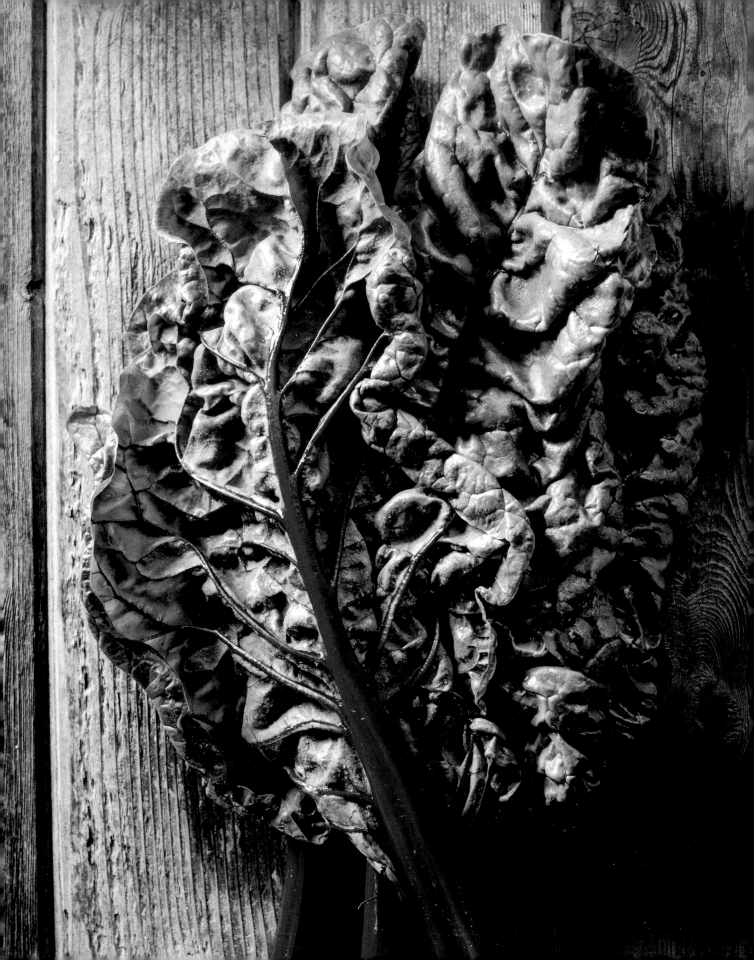

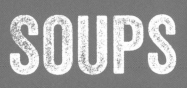

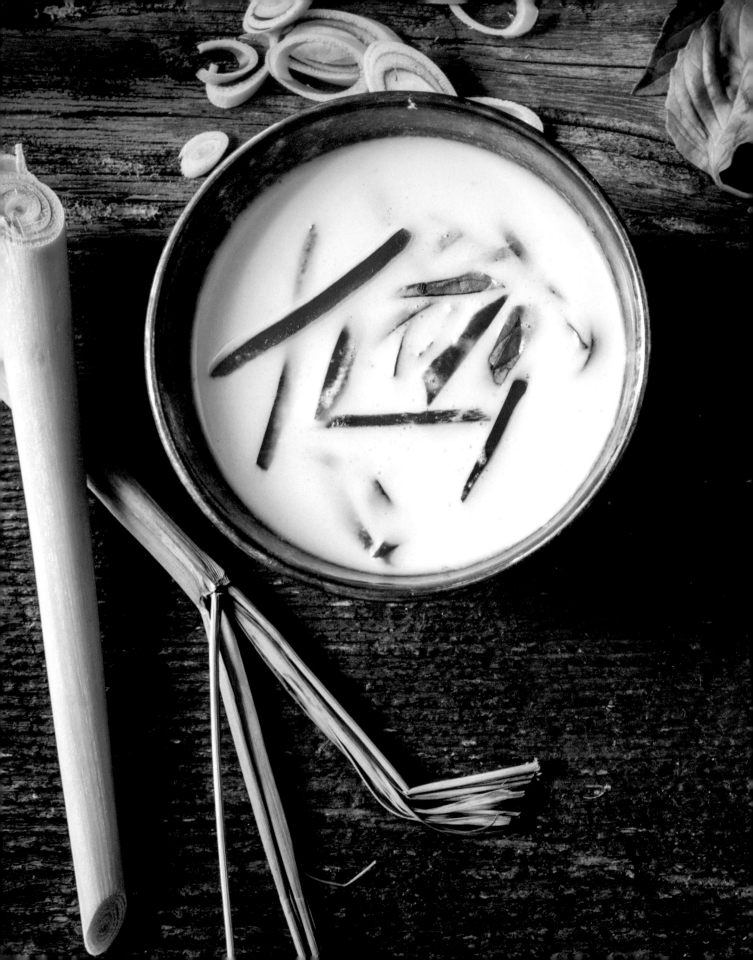

COCONUT, LEMONGRASS & LIME SOUP

This fragrant soup with Thai aromatics and flavors combines nutrient-dense shiitake mushrooms and red bell peppers. Serves 6 to 8

GF Gluten-Free   **SND** Super Nutrient-Dense

Prep Time: 20 minutes

1 tbsp (30 mL) sesame oil

1 tbsp (30 mL) olive oil

2 cloves garlic, minced

½ red onion, finely chopped

1 tbsp (30 mL) fresh ginger, chopped

1 celery stalk, finely chopped

1 cup (250 mL) shiitake mushrooms, sliced thinly

1½ cups (375 mL) vegetable broth

2 cans (14 oz/400 mL each) coconut milk

2 small red chili peppers, minced

1 fresh lemongrass stalk left whole, top cut off and pounded to release aromatics and flavors

1 fresh lemongrass stalk, top cut off and thinly sliced

Small handful of Thai basil leaves

Juice from 1 lime

Sea salt and fresh ground pepper

½ cup (125 mL) red bell peppers, julienned

Heat up the sesame and olive oil in a large pot and sauté the garlic, onion, ginger, celery, and mushrooms until translucent, about 4 to 6 minutes. Add the vegetable broth, coconut milk, chili peppers, and lemongrass stalks. Allow to simmer over low heat for at least 10 minutes. Add salt and pepper to taste. Add the Thai basil leaves and lime juice and serve garnished with julienned red bell peppers.

CHILLED WATERMELON THAI BASIL SOUP

Loaded with electrolytes, this cold soup is fresh and refreshing, making it a summer favorite. Serves 6

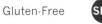 Gluten-Free · · · · SND Super Nutrient-Dense

---

Prep Time: 15 minutes • Special Equipment: blender, fine-mesh sieve

1 medium watermelon, peeled and chopped

1 tbsp agave nectar (optional)

½ cup (125 mL) freshly squeezed lime juice

8 to 10 fresh sweet basil leaves, torn

8 to 10 fresh mint leaves, torn

4 handfuls of sunflower sprouts

½ cup (125 mL) enoki mushrooms

In a blender, blend the watermelon and agave (if using) until smooth. (You may have to do this in batches, depending how large your blender jug is.) Pour through a fine-mesh sieve set over a large bowl. Discard solids.

To the watermelon juice, add the lime juice, basil, and mint. Stir well. Refrigerate until cold, about 1 hour. Serve garnished with sunflower sprouts and enoki mushrooms.

CHIPOTLE CORN CHOWDER

A fresh, spicy, vegetable-packed chowder with rich warmth—a perfect Thrive Energy soup. Serves 8

GF Gluten-Free

Prep Time: 35 minutes • **Special Equipment:** immersion blender or blender

Heat the coconut oil in a large pot over medium-high heat. Add the onions, carrots, celery, garlic, and salt to taste. Cook, stirring occasionally, until onions are translucent.

Stir in the potatoes. Season with salt and pepper to taste. Cook, stirring occasionally, for another 6 or 7 minutes. Stir in the corn and chipotle. Add the vegetable stock, coconut milk, and bouillon cubes. Increase heat to high and bring to a boil. As soon as it starts boiling, reduce heat to a simmer. Simmer soup for 15 to 20 minutes, until carrots and potatoes are fork-tender. Remove from heat.

Using an immersion blender or blender, purée the soup just a little, keeping the texture somewhat chunky. Adjust seasoning and stir in chives and parsley. Serve garnished with the cilantro and red peppers.

¼ cup (60 mL) coconut oil

2 cups (500 mL) diced onions

1 cup (250 mL) diced carrots

1 cup (250 mL) diced celery

3 or 4 cloves garlic, minced

Sea salt and freshly ground black pepper to taste

2 to 3 large red potatoes, peeled and diced

5 cups (1.25 L) fresh sweet corn kernels (from about 10 cobs)

2 to 3 tbsp (30 to 45 mL) minced chipotle pepper in adobo sauce, or to taste

6 cups (1.5 L) vegetable stock

2 cups (500 mL) coconut milk

2 to 3 vegan vegetable bouillon cubes

1 bunch chives, chopped

Small handful of fresh parsley, chopped

Chopped fresh cilantro, for garnish

½ cup (125 mL) red bell peppers, julienned, for garnish

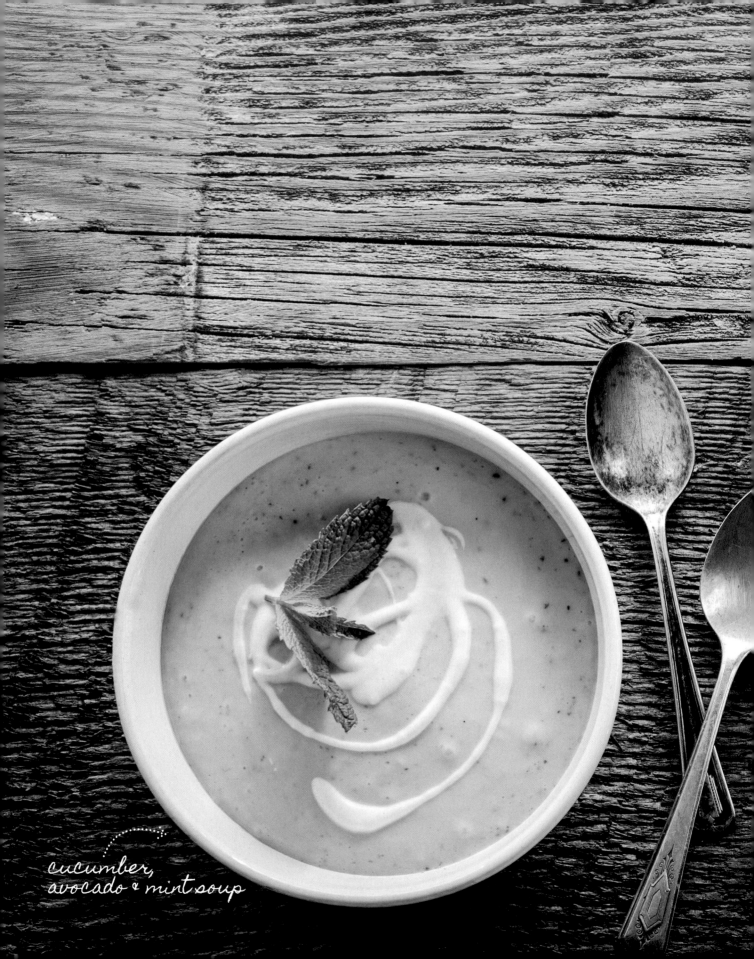

cucumber,
avocado & mint soup

carrot, avocado
& coconut soup

CARROT, AVOCADO & COCONUT SOUP

With an innovative combination of complementary flavors, this soup is also mineral-rich and alkaline-forming. Serves 6

 GF Gluten-Free

Prep Time: 20 minutes • **Special Equipment:** high-speed juice extractor, blender

1 ripe avocado, peeled

1 small clove garlic, chopped

4 medium carrots, peeled and juiced

4 cups (1 L) coconut milk

2 tsp (10 mL) freshly squeezed lime juice

1 tsp (5 mL) yellow curry paste

Small handful of fresh cilantro leaves, torn

Sea salt and freshly ground black pepper

½ cup (125 mL) roasted cashews, coarsely chopped

In a blender, combine the avocado, garlic, carrot juice, coconut milk, lime juice, curry paste, half of the cilantro leaves, and salt and pepper to taste. Blend until smooth. Serve garnished with cashews and the remaining cilantro leaves.

CUCUMBER, AVOCADO & MINT SOUP

A fresh tasting, simple, wholesome creamy soup is ideal in the warmer months.
Serves 6

 Gluten-Free

Prep Time: 10 minutes • **Special Equipment:** citrus juicer, blender

Combine cucumber, avocado, lime juice, garlic, ¾ of the mint, cumin, cilantro, pepper, and sea salt in blender and purée. Add coconut milk and lightly blend, adjusting salt if needed. Serve chilled in bowls and top with a pinch of chili powder and green onions. Garnish with a sprig of fresh mint.

· ·

• Drizzle with some coconut milk for a beautiful contrast.

3 medium peeled cucumbers, coarsely chopped

1 ripe avocado, peeled

¼ cup (60 mL) freshly squeezed lime juice

1 small clove garlic, chopped

Small handful of fresh mint leaves, torn, leaving some for garnish

½ tsp (2 mL) cumin powder

Small handful of fresh cilantro leaves, torn

¼ tsp (1 mL) freshly ground black pepper

½ tsp (2 mL) sea salt

1 cup (250 mL) coconut milk

Pinch of chili powder

1 tsp (5 mL) green onion, for garnish

Fresh mint leaves, for garnish

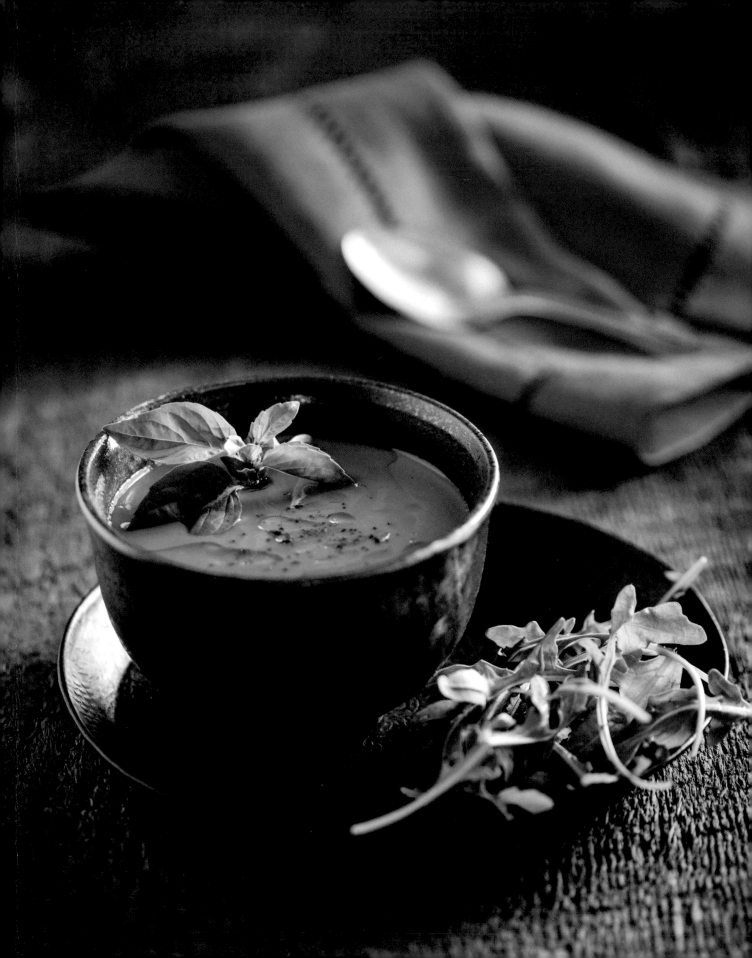

ROASTED RED PEPPER & SWEET POTATO SOUP

Well-balanced flavor and clean carbohydrate make this soup a delicious, functional favorite. Serves 6 to 8

GF Gluten-Free   **SND** Super Nutrient-Dense

Prep Time: 25 minutes • **Special Equipment:** immersion blender or blender

Preheat oven to 375°F (190°C).

Place the sweet potatoes and the onions on a baking sheet. Drizzle with a little of the grapeseed oil. Season with salt and pepper to taste. Toss to coat. Roast for 20 minutes or until golden. Set aside.

Heat the remaining grapeseed oil in a stockpot over medium-high heat. Add the celery, carrots, garlic, and salt to taste. Stir in the roasted peppers and sweet potato mixture and cook on medium for 10 minutes.

Add the vegetable stock and coconut milk. Season with salt and pepper. Increase heat to high and bring to a boil. As soon as it starts boiling, reduce heat to a simmer. Simmer soup, uncovered, for 15 to 20 minutes. Remove from heat.

Using an immersion blender or blender, purée the soup to the desired consistency. Adjust seasoning. Stir in most of the basil, reserving a few leaves for garnish. Adjust seasoning. Serve garnished with the remaining basil leaves.

2 large sweet potatoes, peeled and cubed

1 cup (250 mL) chopped onions

¼ cup (60 mL) grapeseed oil

Sea salt and freshly ground black pepper

1 cup (250 mL) chopped celery

1 cup (250 mL) chopped carrots

3 or 4 cloves garlic, minced

4 large roasted red peppers, coarsely chopped

4 to 5 cups (1 to 1.25 L) vegetable stock

1 cup (250 mL) coconut milk

Large handful of fresh sweet basil, thinly sliced

SPICY MISO MUSHROOM SOUP

Asian-inspired and mineral-rich, this alkalizing soup is bursting with classic flavors.
Serves 6

GF Gluten-Free   **SND** Super Nutrient-Dense

Prep Time: 15 minutes

¼ cup (60 mL) virgin coconut oil

2 cups (500 mL) diced sweet onions

1 cup (250 mL) diced leeks

1 cup (250 mL) diced celery

Sea salt and freshly ground black pepper to taste

2 Thai red chilies, seeded if desired, finely chopped

3 or 4 cloves garlic, finely chopped

2 tbsp (30 mL) freshly squeezed lime juice

2 tbsp (30 mL) miso paste

1 tbsp (15 mL) ground cumin

1 tbsp (15 mL) ground coriander

1 tbsp (15 mL) paprika

4 cups (1 L) diced king oyster mushrooms

2 cups (500 mL) enoki mushrooms, cut in half crosswise

6 to 8 cups (1.5 to 2 L) vegetable stock

2 to 3 vegan vegetable bouillon cubes

1 tsp (5 mL) Sriracha sauce, or to taste (optional)

3 green onions, finely chopped, for garnish

½ cup (125 mL) bean sprouts, for garnish

Heat the coconut oil in a stockpot over medium-high heat. Add the onions, leeks, celery, and salt to taste. Cook, stirring occasionally, until onions are translucent.

Stir in the chilies, garlic, lime juice, and miso paste. Add cumin, coriander, paprika, and salt and pepper to taste. Add the king oyster mushrooms and enoki mushrooms. Cook, stirring frequently, until the mushrooms are tender and have released some of their juices, about 3 minutes.

Add the vegetable stock and bouillon cubes. Increase heat to high and bring to a boil. As soon as it starts boiling, reduce heat to a simmer. Stir in Sriracha sauce (if using) and simmer for 15 minutes. Adjust seasoning, adding more lime juice, Sriracha, and/or salt until you reach a balance of acid and heat. Serve garnished with green onions and bean sprouts.

SWEET POTATO, BLACK BEAN & SWEET CORN CHILI

This satisfying southwestern chili is sure to please those with a hearty appetite.
Serves 6

GF Gluten-Free (Option)

Prep Time: 30 minutes

3 cups (750 mL) cubed sweet potatoes

4 tbsp (60 mL) virgin coconut oil

1 cup (250 mL) chopped sweet onions

4 tbsp (60 mL) minced garlic

¼ cup (60 mL) chili powder

3 tbsp (45 mL) ground cumin

3 cups (750 mL) vine-ripened tomatoes, quartered

3 cups (750 mL) sweet corn kernels

2 cans (14 oz/400 g each) black beans, drained and rinsed

Large handful of fresh cilantro leaves

½ cup (125 mL) lime juice

1 to 2 jalapeño peppers, seeded and finely chopped

1 cup (250 mL) vegetable stock

4 slices sprouted bread (my favorite is Silver Hills)

Sea salt and freshly ground black pepper

3 cups (750 mL) shredded Daiya or your favorite dairy-free Cheddar-style cheese, or Cheddar cashew cheese (page 24)

¾ cup (175 mL) cashew sour cream (page 68)

½ cup (125 mL) finely chopped chives, for garnish

In a large saucepan, cover the sweet potatoes with salted water. Bring to a boil and boil until they are slightly undercooked. Drain, then transfer to a bowl of ice water to stop the cooking. Drain again.

In a medium saucepan, heat 2 tbsp (30 mL) of the coconut oil over medium heat. Add the onions and 2 tbsp (30 mL) of the garlic. Sweat, stirring occasionally, until onions are translucent.

Stir in the chili powder and cumin; cook for 2 minutes. Add the sweet potatoes, tomatoes, corn, beans, cilantro, lime juice, and most of the jalapeños, reserving some for garnish. Simmer, uncovered, over medium-low heat for 30 minutes. If the chili is too thick, add the vegetable stock until desired consistency is achieved.

About 10 minutes before serving, preheat the broiler. Arrange the bread on a baking sheet. Brush both sides with the remaining 2 tbsp (30 mL) coconut oil, then rub the top of each slice with a small pinch of the remaining garlic. Broil until golden brown. Cut each slice in half diagonally.

Season the chili with salt and pepper to taste.

Top each serving with ½ cup (125 mL) of the cheese and 2 tbsp (30 mL) sour cream. Garnish with chives and remaining jalapeño. Serve with garlic bread on the side.

ROASTED SWEET POTATO, CARROT & GINGER SOUP

An autumn favorite, this mineral-rich and satisfying soup lets the earthy natural flavors of root vegetables shine. **Serves 6**

 GF Gluten-Free

Prep Time: 25 minutes • **Special Equipment:** immersion blender or blender

3 large sweet potatoes, peeled and cubed

6 or 7 cloves garlic, peeled

1 cup (250 mL) leeks, chopped

5 large carrots, peeled and cubed

2 cups (500 mL) chopped sweet onions

¼ cup (60 mL) grapeseed oil

Sea salt and freshly ground black pepper to taste

6 to 8 thyme stems

1 cup (250 mL) chopped celery

2-inch (5 cm) knob of fresh ginger, peeled and chopped

½ tsp (2 mL) nutmeg

2 cups (500 mL) coconut milk

4 to 6 cups (1 to 1.5 L) vegetable stock

2 to 3 vegan vegetable bouillon cubes

Small handful of fresh thyme leaves

Preheat oven to 375°F (190°C).

Place the sweet potatoes, garlic, leeks, carrots, and half of the onions on a baking sheet. Drizzle with half of the grapeseed oil and season with salt and pepper. Toss to coat. Place thyme stems randomly on the vegetables. Roast, stirring once halfway through, for 20 minutes or until potatoes and carrots are golden and tender. Discard thyme stems.

Heat the remaining grapeseed oil in a stockpot over medium-high heat. Add celery, remaining onions, and salt to taste. Cook, stirring occasionally, until onions are translucent.

Stir in the roasted vegetables, ginger, and nutmeg. Add the coconut milk, reserving 2 tbsp (15 mL) for garnish, if desired. Bring to a simmer. Stir in the vegetable stock and bouillon cubes. Season with salt and pepper to taste. Simmer on medium heat for 15 to 20 minutes. Remove from heat.

Using an immersion blender or blender, purée the soup to desired consistency. Adjust seasoning. Stir in most of the fresh thyme, reserving some for garnish.

Drizzle each serving with reserved coconut milk (if using) and sprinkle with remaining thyme leaves.

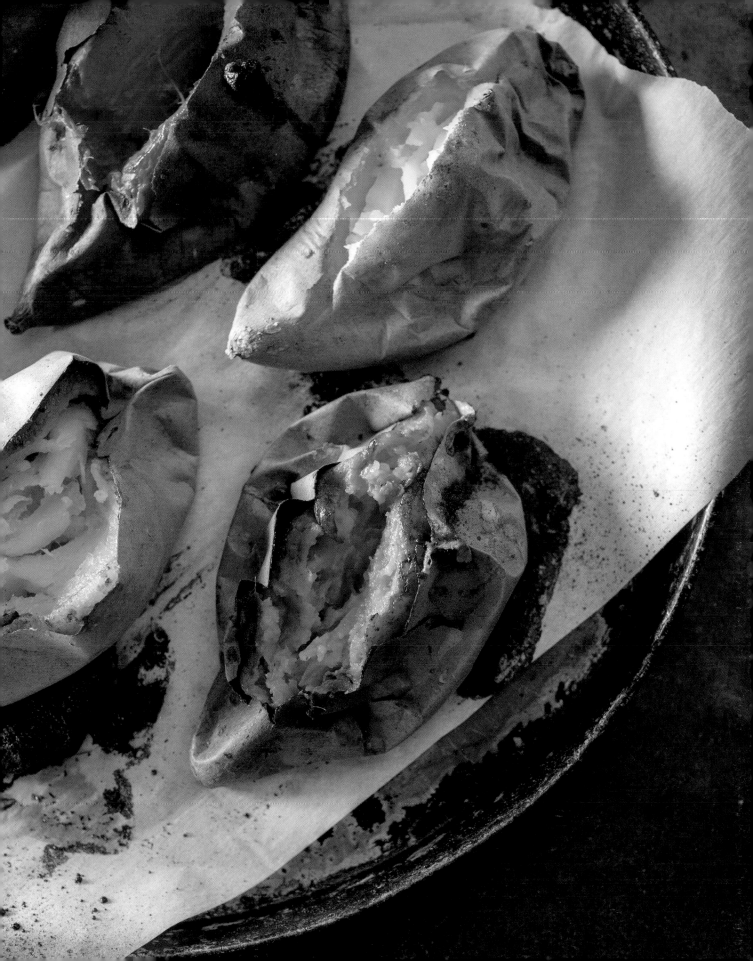

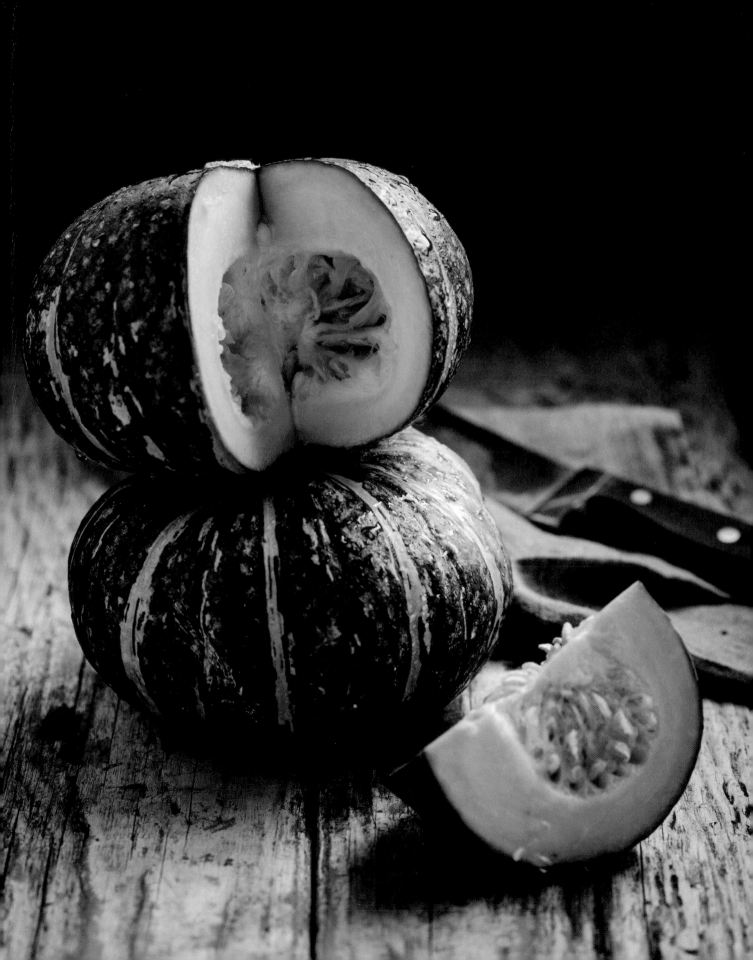

ROASTED FENNEL, SQUASH & RED POTATO STEW WITH RED CABBAGE SALAD

A hearty autumn favorite, this stew will stick to your ribs without causing an energy crash. Serves 4

 Gluten-Free   **SND** Super Nutrient-Dense

Prep Time: 25 minutes

For the stew, preheat oven to 350°F (180°C). In a large bowl, toss fennel, squash, carrots, garlic, onions, and red potatoes with the oil. Spread in a single layer on a baking sheet. Randomly place the thyme on the vegetables. Roast, stirring once halfway through, until fork-tender, 30 to 40 minutes.

Heat the stock in a large saucepan. Add the roasted vegetables and simmer for 25 to 30 minutes. Season to taste with sea salt and pepper.

While the stew simmers, make the red cabbage salad. In a medium bowl, combine the thyme and red wine vinegar. Add the oil in a slow stream, whisking until emulsified. Add the cabbage and mix well, coating the cabbage with the vinaigrette. Set aside for 15 minutes. Season to taste with sea salt and pepper.

Serve the stew topped with the salad and garnished with parsley.

Stew

2 cups (500 mL) chopped fennel

2 cups (500 mL) peeled and chopped butternut squash

2 cups (500 mL) chopped carrots

6 to 8 whole garlic cloves

2 cups (500 mL) chopped red onions

2 cups (500 mL) chopped red potatoes

¼ cup (60 mL) grapeseed oil

6 to 8 thyme stems

4 cups (1 L) vegetable stock

Sea salt and freshly ground black pepper

Large handful of fresh parsley leaves, torn, for garnish

Red Cabbage Salad

Leaves from 4 sprigs thyme, finely chopped

½ cup (125 mL) red wine vinegar

¼ cup (60 mL) grapeseed oil

2 cups (500 mL) thinly sliced red cabbage

Sea salt and freshly ground black pepper

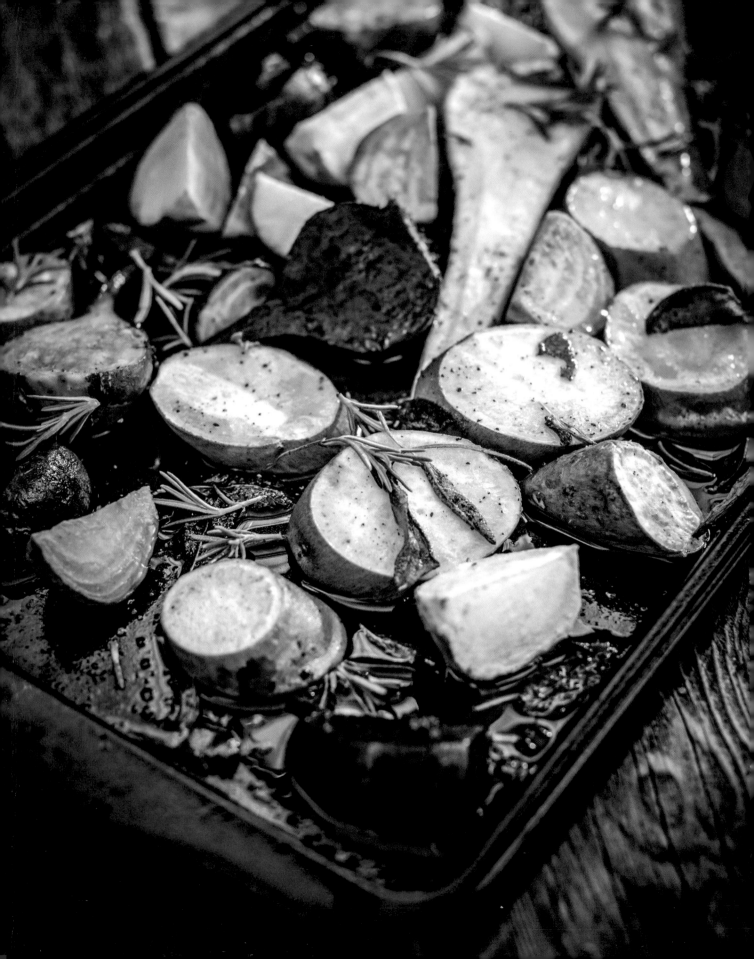

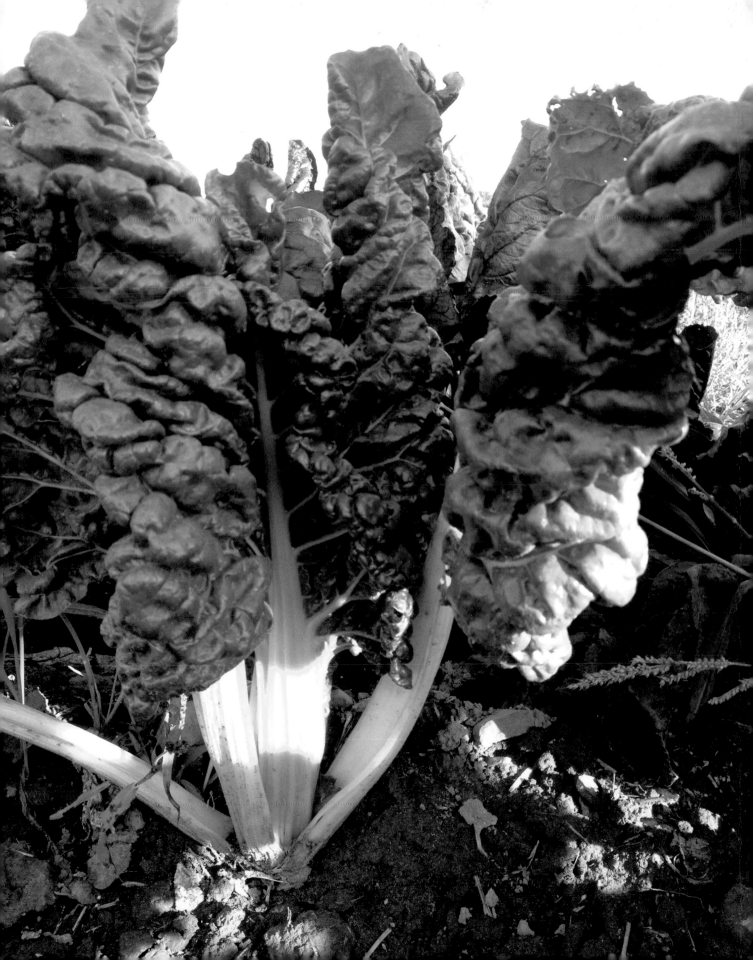

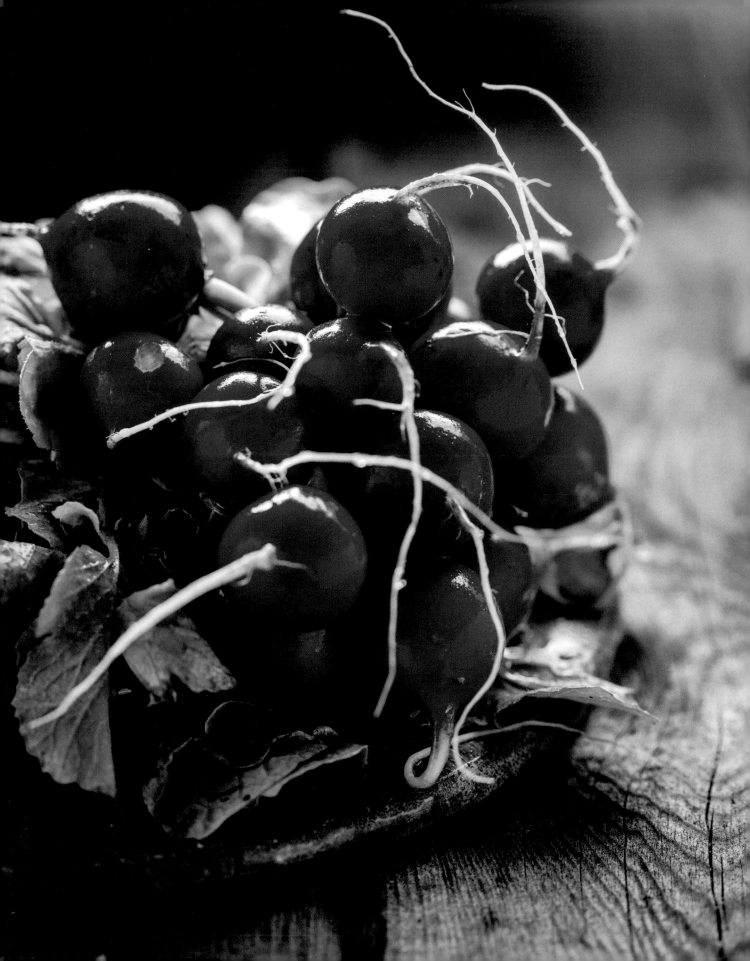

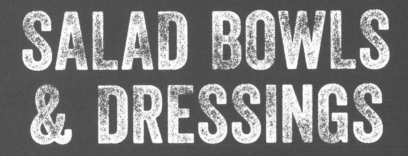

SALAD BOWLS
& DRESSINGS

ASIAN JULIENNED VEGETABLE MIX

A good staple to have on hand, this recipe is packed with a variety of vegetables, and therefore is exceptionally nutrient-dense. Using a mandoline to julienne the vegetables saves a lot of time. Makes 6 cups (1.5 L)

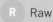 Raw   GF Gluten-Free   SND Super Nutrient-Dense

---

Prep Time: 10 minutes
Special Equipment: mandoline with julienne blade or julienne peeler

2 cups (500 mL) thinly sliced savoy or napa cabbage

1 cup (250 mL) thinly sliced red cabbage

1 cup (250 mL) peeled and julienned carrots

1 cup (250 mL) peeled and julienned daikon

1 cup (250 mL) julienned baby bok choy

In a large bowl, toss all the ingredients together.

• Keeps in a sealed container, refrigerated, for up to 5 days.

BIG GREEN SALAD

Full of chlorophyll with its variety of lettuces and sprouts, this is one of the most nutrient-dense Thrive Energy salads. This one is for those who appreciate greens, and a lot of them! Serves 1

R Raw   **GF** Gluten-Free   **SND** Super Nutrient-Dense

Prep Time: 15 minutes

In a large serving bowl, toss together the spring mix and spinach. Top with the sprouts, sugar snap peas, cucumber, hemp hearts, sunflower seeds, and croutons.

Fan out the avocado on top of the salad. Drizzle with the cucumber avocado dressing. Scatter the jalapeño over the top and drizzle with the hemp oil.

....

• For a great variation, add 3 falafels (page 67).

Large handful of spring mix greens

Small handful of baby spinach

1 cup (250 mL) sunflower sprouts

½ cup (125 mL) sugar snap peas, trimmed and thinly sliced lengthwise

½ cup (125 mL) diced cucumber

2 tbsp (30 mL) hemp hearts

2 tbsp (30 mL) sunflower seeds

Small handful of garlic oregano croutons (page 144)

1 avocado, peeled and thinly sliced

½ cup (125 mL) cucumber avocado dressing (page 145)

1 tsp (5 mL) finely chopped jalapeño pepper

Drizzle of hemp oil

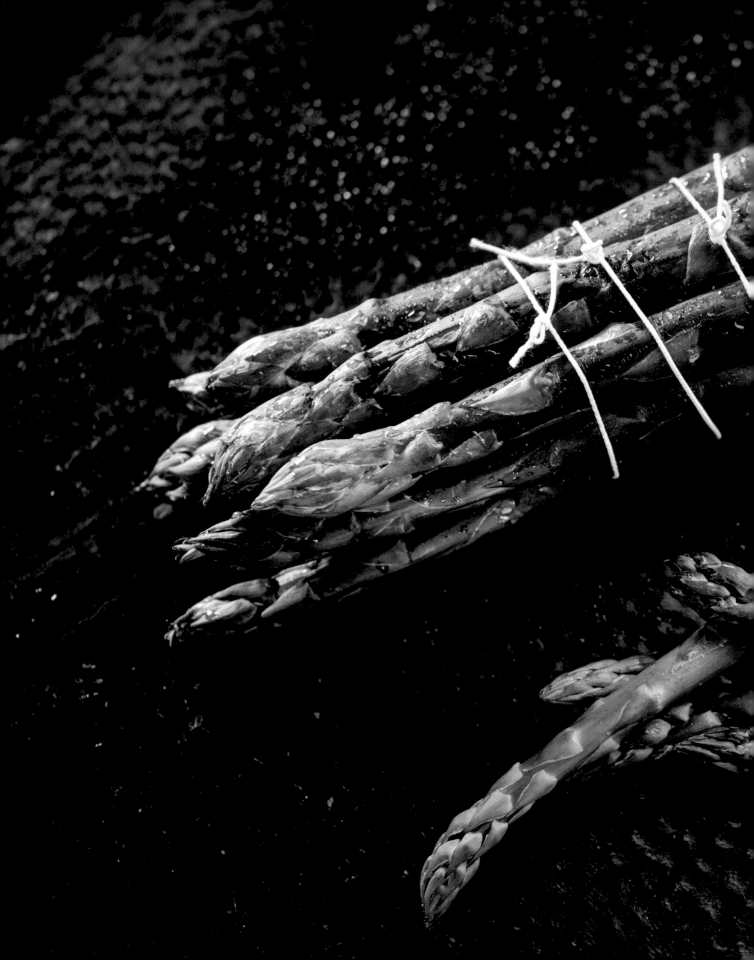

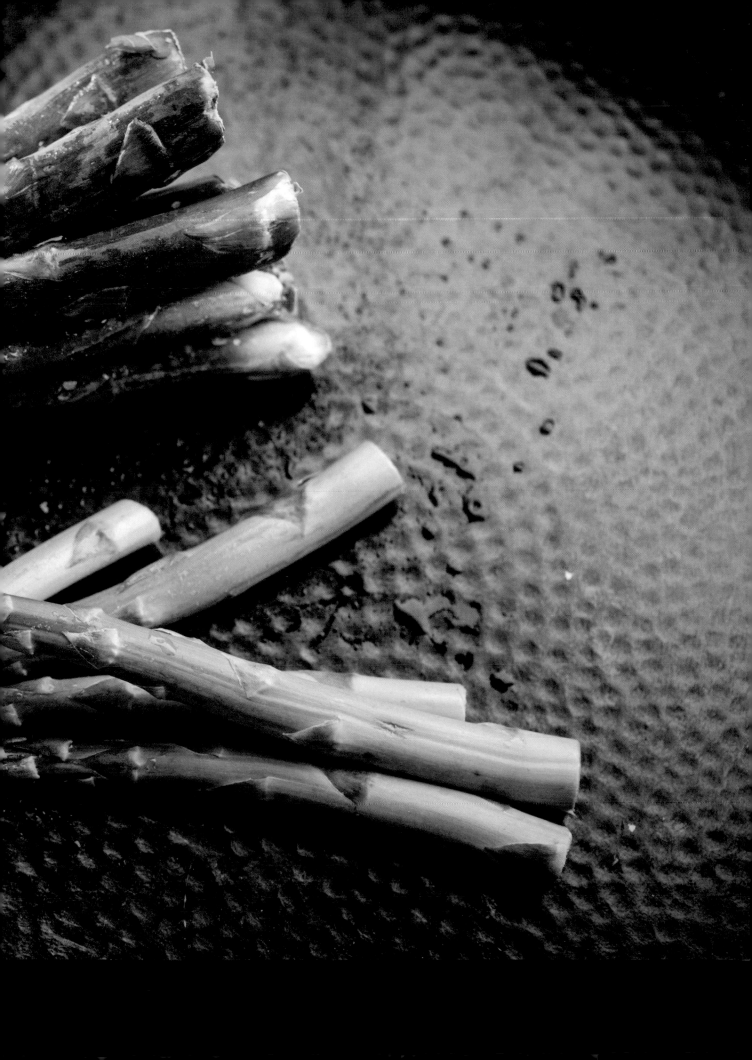

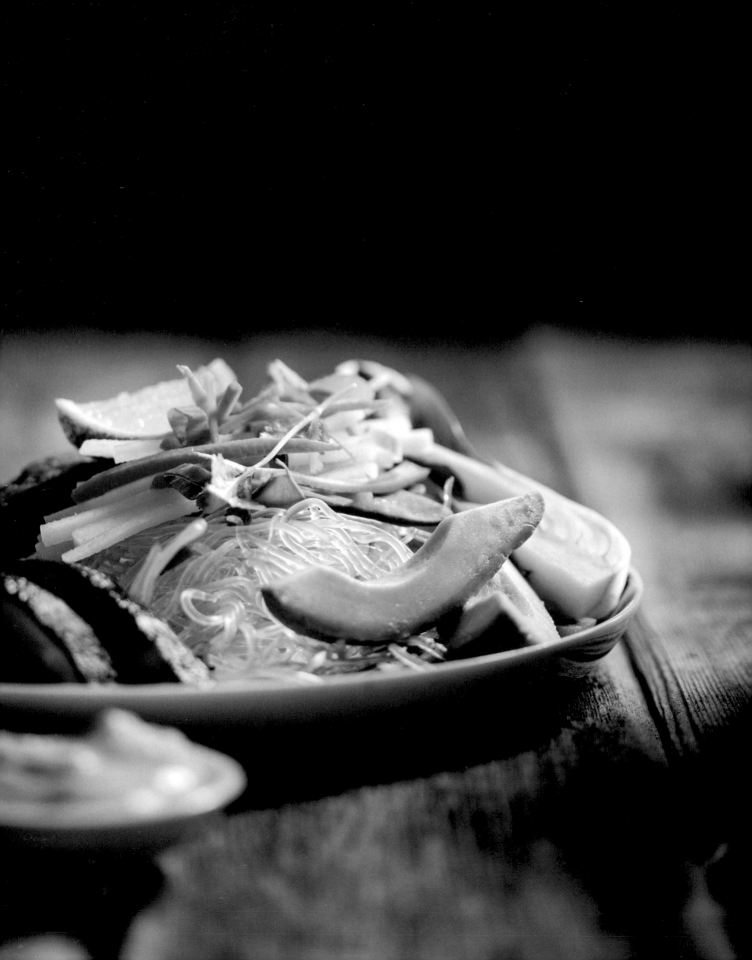

AVOCADO & KELP NOODLE SALAD

The kelp and miso add plenty of minerals along with Asian flavor. Serves 1

 R Raw   **GF** Gluten-Free   **SND** Super Nutrient-Dense

Prep Time: 15 minutes • **Special Equipment:** blender, fine-mesh sieve

In a large bowl, combine the spinach, kelp noodles, red cabbage, and some of the sesame seeds. Add the vinaigrette and toss, making sure all the ingredients are covered. Add the avocado and toss lightly. Season with salt and pepper to taste (if using).

On one end of a rectangular plate, place a dollop of the wasabi aïoli. Using tongs, pile the salad mix on the other side of the plate. Try to achieve height while plating the salad. Sprinkle the salad with the basil and remaining sesame seeds. Garnish with nori and lime wedge.

....

• Take a small dab of aïoli with every bite for a burst of flavor.

Handful of baby spinach

1 cup (250 mL) raw kelp noodles, rinsed

½ cup (125 mL) thinly sliced red cabbage

Few pinches of white sesame seeds

About ⅓ to ½ cup (75 to 125 mL) sesame, ginger & white miso vinaigrette (page 147)

½ ripe avocado, peeled and chopped

Sea salt and freshly ground black pepper (optional)

1 dollop wasabi aïoli (page 79)

4 or 5 fresh Thai basil leaves, thinly sliced

¼ cup (60 mL) julienned nori

Lime wedge, for garnish

BABY ARUGULA, RED BEET & ASIAN PEAR SALAD

Beets are packed with nitrates, which convert into nitrous oxide that helps enhance oxygen utilization, so this salad is ideal for people who are physically active. The flavors are fresh and naturally sweet. Serves 1 or 2

 Raw Gluten-Free **SND** Super Nutrient-Dense

Prep Time: 15 minutes
Special Equipment: mandoline with julienne blade or julienne peeler

Large handful of baby arugula

Large handful of frisée leaves, coarsely chopped

½ medium Asian or Bartlett pear, cut in half, cored, and thinly shaved

¼ to ⅓ cup (60 to 75 mL) raspberry & sweet basil balsamic vinaigrette (page 147)

Sea salt and freshly ground black pepper

1 medium red beet (unpeeled), julienned

¼ cup (60 mL) walnuts, coarsely chopped

In a medium bowl, combine the arugula, frisée, and half of the shaved pears. Add the vinaigrette and toss gently to coat. Season with salt and pepper to taste.

Transfer the salad to a serving bowl or plates and top with the red beets and walnuts. Scatter with the remaining pear slices. Serve immediately.

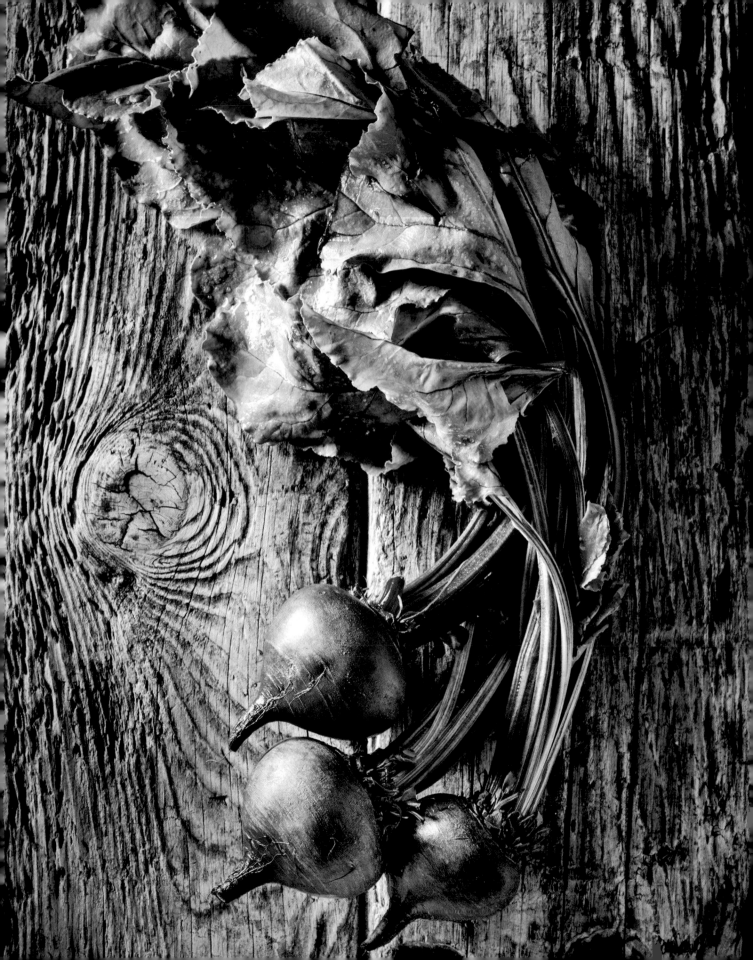

GINGER, LEMONGRASS & PEANUT SALAD

The fresh, citrusy flavors in this salad are perfect on a summer day. This salad reduces inflammation and improves digestion. It can be a meal in itself. Serves 1

GF Gluten-Free   **SND** Super Nutrient-Dense

Prep Time: 12 minutes
Special Equipment: mandoline with julienne blade or julienne peeler

Large handful of spring mix greens

Handful of Asian julienned vegetable mix (page 128)

3 to 4 tbsp (45 to 60 mL) pad Thai sauce (page 76)

1 tbsp (15 mL) ginger & lemongrass vinaigrette (page 146)

⅓ cup (75 mL) bean sprouts

5 or 6 snow peas, trimmed and thinly sliced lengthwise

⅓ cup (75 mL) peeled and julienned watermelon radish

3 slices sesame garlic tempeh, grilled on each side for 2 to 3 minutes (optional)

3 to 4 tbsp (45 to 60 mL) chopped toasted peanuts

Small handful pea shoots, for garnish

1 tsp (5 mL) sesame oil

Lime wedge, for garnish

In a medium bowl, combine the spring mix, Asian vegetable mix, pad Thai sauce, and vinaigrette. Toss gently until everything is lightly coated.

In a large serving bowl, layer the salad with the bean sprouts, snow peas, and watermelon radish.

Stack the tempeh slices (if using) and slice diagonally. Place to one side of the salad. Sprinkle the salad with the peanuts and garnish with the pea shoots. Drizzle with sesame oil and garnish with a lime wedge.

....

• I prefer sesame garlic marinated tempeh from Turtle Island Foods.

WATERMELON, CUCUMBER & STRAWBERRY SALAD

A summertime favorite packed with hydrating and antioxidant qualities.

Serves 1 or 2

GF Gluten-Free   **SND** Super Nutrient-Dense

Prep Time: 6 to 8 minutes • **Special Equipment:** mandoline

In a medium bowl, whisk together the mint, lime juice, grapeseed oil, and agave nectar. Add the watermelon, cucumber, strawberries, and fennel. Gently fold to coat. Season to taste with sea salt and pepper.

. . . .

• Don't throw out the fennel fronds. They taste fresh and make an attractive garnish.

Small handful of fresh mint leaves, torn

2 tbsp (30 mL) freshly squeezed lime juice

2 tbsp (30 mL) grapeseed oil

1 tsp (5 mL) agave nectar

1 cup (250 mL) watermelon cut in bite-size pieces

1 cup (250 mL) English cucumber cut in bite-size pieces

½ cup (125 mL) fresh strawberries, sliced

¼ cup (60 mL) thinly shaved fennel

Coarse sea salt and a pinch of freshly ground black pepper

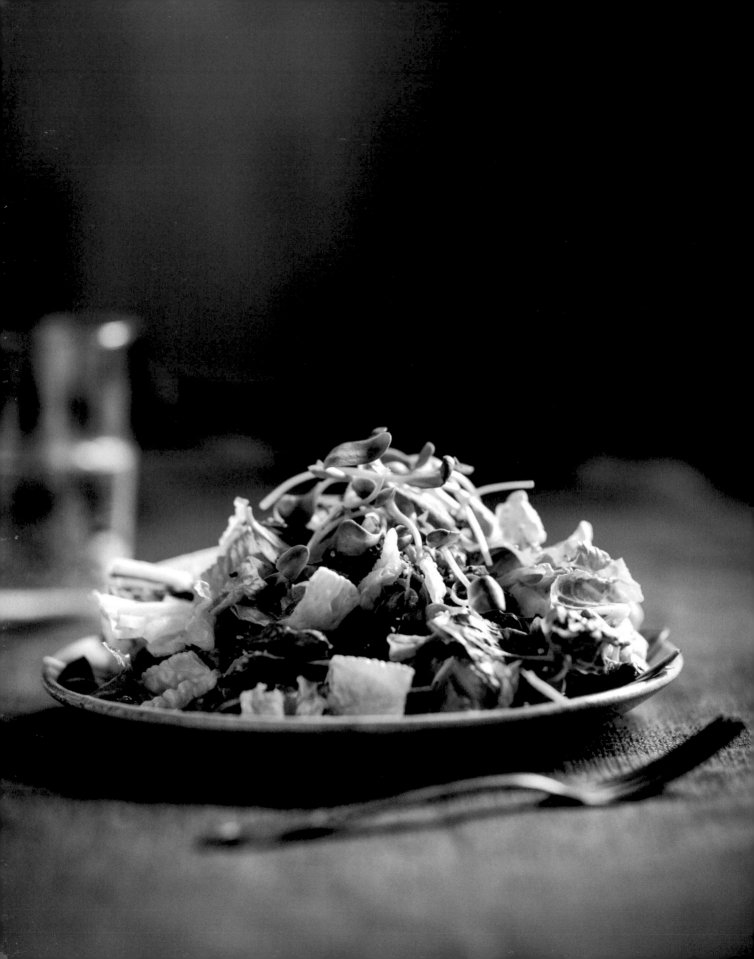

CAESAR SPROUT SALAD

Crispy and rich like a traditional Caesar salad but with all the functional benefits of nutrient-dense plant-based ingredients. This is an ideal transitional salad for those who are progressing to a plant-based diet. Serves 1

R Raw **GF** Gluten-Free **SND** Super Nutrient-Dense

Prep Time: 10 minutes • **Special Equipment:** grill pan

In a large bowl, combine the spinach, romaine hearts, and cucumber. Add the Caesar dressing and toss to coat.

Transfer the salad to a serving bowl and top with the sprouts and croutons.

Stack the tempeh slices (if using) and julienne diagonally. Place to one side of the salad. Drizzle salad with avocado oil and garnish with capers.

· ·

• I prefer smoky maple marinated tempeh from Turtle Island Foods.

Handful of baby spinach

3 cups (750 mL) coarsely chopped romaine hearts

½ cup (125 mL) peeled and diced English cucumber

⅓ to ½ cup (75 to 125 mL) vegan Caesar salad dressing

Handful of sunflower sprouts

⅓ cup (75 mL) garlic oregano croutons (page 144)

3 slices smoky maple tempeh, grilled on each side for 2 to 3 minutes (optional)

Drizzle of avocado oil

1 tbsp (15 mL) capers, for garnish

GRILLED POTATO SALAD

A meal fit for a lumberjack, yet pleasantly fresh. It can easily be turned into a transition meal to help those progressing from standard meals to clean, plant-based ones. Serves 3 or 4

 Transition   GF Gluten-Free

Prep Time: 12 minutes • **Special Equipment:** grill pan

2 lb (900 g) fingerling red or mixed colored potatoes (15 to 20)

¼ cup (60 mL) virgin coconut oil, melted

Sea salt and freshly ground black pepper

⅓ cup (75 mL) roasted garlic aïoli (page 78)

1 tbsp (15 mL) agave nectar

2 tsp (10 mL) red wine vinegar

2 tsp (10 mL) freshly squeezed lemon juice

Small handful of baby spinach

2 tbsp (30 mL) chopped fresh parsley

2 slices smoky maple tempeh, grilled on each side for 2 to 3 minutes (optional)

1 green onion, finely chopped

¼ cup (60 mL) shredded Daiya or your favorite dairy-free Cheddar-style cheese (transition option), or Cheddar cashew cheese (page 24)

In a large saucepan, cover the potatoes with water. Add a few pinches of salt and bring to a boil. Reduce heat and simmer until tender, about 15 minutes. Drain and let cool. Cut the potatoes in half lengthwise.

Heat a grill pan over medium-high heat. Brush the potatoes with coconut oil and season to taste with salt and pepper. Grill the potatoes for 5 minutes per side or until they have light grill marks.

In a large bowl, stir together the aïoli, agave, red wine vinegar, and lemon juice. Add the potatoes, spinach, and half of the parsley. Toss well. Transfer to a serving bowl.

Stack the tempeh slices (if using) and slice diagonally. Top the salad with the green onions, tempeh, cheese, and remaining parsley.

....

• I prefer smoky maple marinated tempeh from Turtle Island Foods.

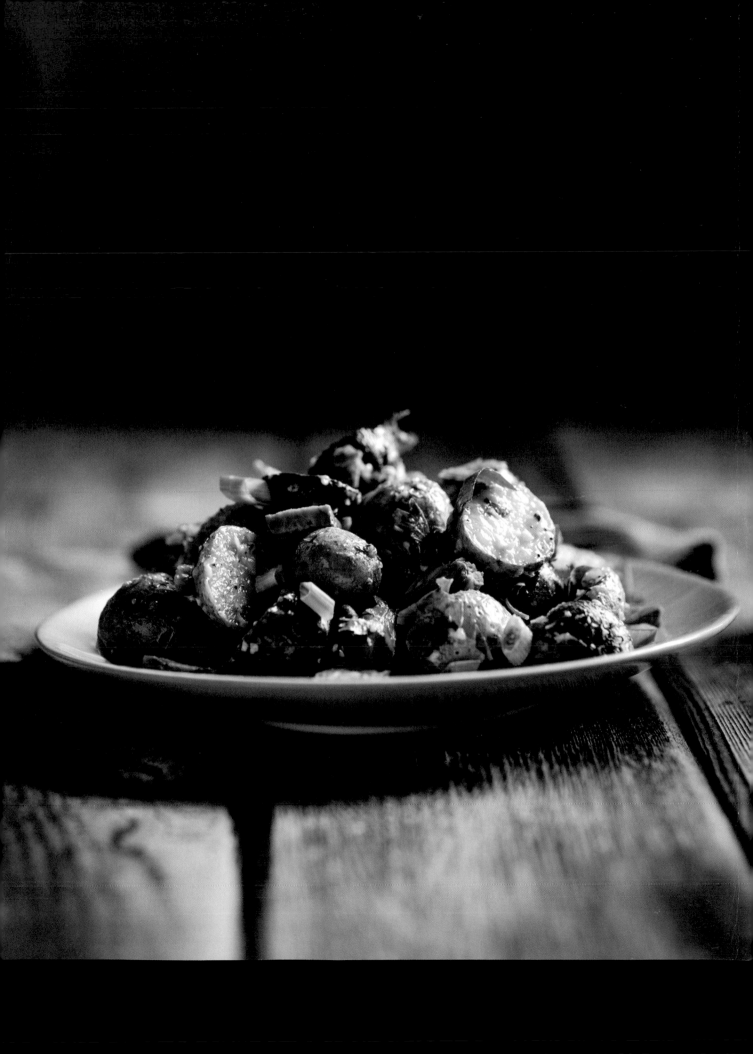

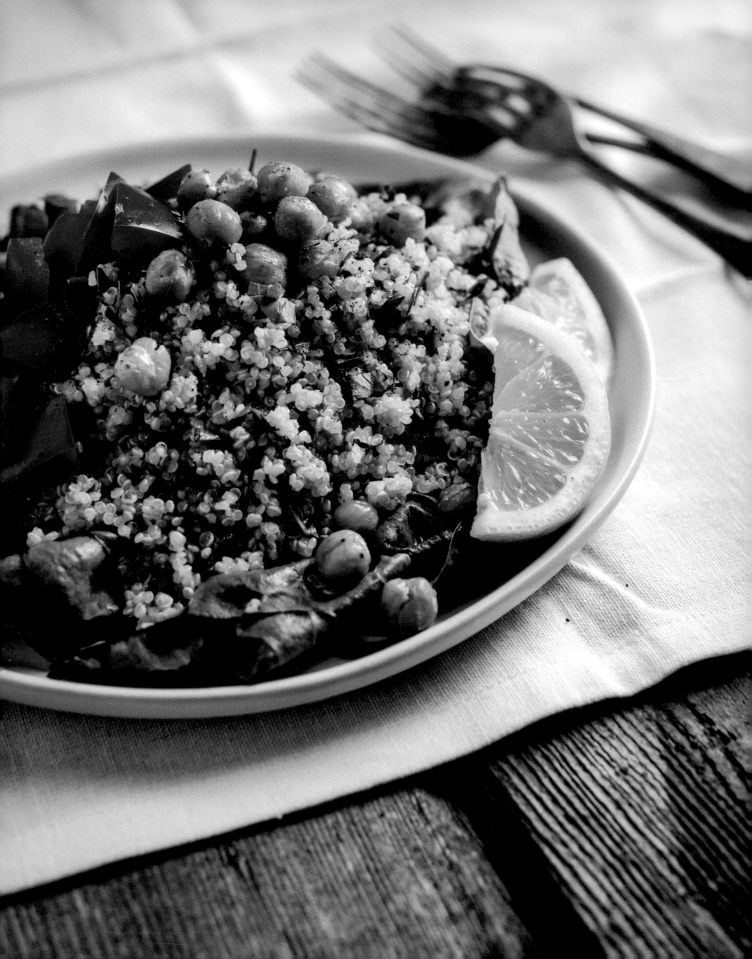

QUINOA TABBOULEH SALAD

A gluten-free twist on a traditional recipe, with loads more nutrients. Traditional tabbouleh is made with couscous, which is standard wheat. Quinoa contains about 20 percent more protein, is gluten-free, and is considerably easier to digest than wheat. Serves 2 or 3

GF Gluten-Free   **SND** Super Nutrient-Dense

Prep Time: 18 minutes

¼ cup (60 mL) virgin coconut oil

1 cup (250 mL) quinoa (any color), rinsed and drained

2 cups (500 mL) water

1 large sweet onion, finely chopped

2 tbsp (30 mL) ground cumin

1 tbsp (15 mL) ground coriander

1 tbsp (15 mL) red pepper flakes

1 tbsp (15 mL) tomato paste

1 tbsp (15 mL) Mediterranean red pepper paste

2 medium tomatoes, seeded and diced

6 green onions, finely chopped

5 or 6 fresh mint leaves, torn

1½ cups (375 mL) fresh Italian parsley, chopped

2 tbsp (30 mL) freshly squeezed lemon juice

1 tbsp (15 mL) pomegranate molasses

1 tbsp (15 mL) grapeseed oil

Sea salt and freshly ground black pepper to taste

Lemon wedge, for garnish

Heat a medium saucepan over medium-high heat and drizzle the bottom with some of the virgin coconut oil. Add the quinoa; toast, stirring frequently, for 1 to 2 minutes or until dry. Add the water and bring to a boil. Reduce heat to the lowest setting, cover, and cook for 15 minutes. Remove from heat and let the quinoa sit, covered, for 5 minutes. Fluff with a fork, transfer to a large bowl, and let cool.

Meanwhile, heat another medium saucepan over medium-high heat. Add the remaining coconut oil and the onions. Cook, stirring frequently, until the onions are translucent, 3 to 4 minutes. Add the cumin, coriander, red pepper flakes, tomato paste, and red pepper paste. Cook, stirring, for another 3 to 4 minutes. Let cool.

Add the paste mixture to the quinoa and toss gently until fully incorporated. Add the tomatoes, green onions, mint, parsley, lemon juice, pomegranate molasses, and grapeseed oil. Toss gently. Season with salt and pepper to taste and garnish with lemon wedge.

. . . .

• **Look for Mediterranean red pepper paste in Middle Eastern supermarkets or in the foreign food aisle at the grocery store.**

GARLIC OREGANO CROUTONS

Simple to make and full of flavor, these croutons add sustenance and crunch to any salad. My favorite breads to use are Silver Hills Squirrelly and Mack's Flax. You can also use gluten-free breads. Makes 3 cups (750 mL)

 Gluten-Free (Option)

Prep Time: 5 minutes

3 tbsp (45 mL) grapeseed oil

1 tsp (5 mL) dried oregano

1 tsp (5 mL) garlic powder

Pinch of sea salt

6 slices sprouted bread, crusts removed, cubed

Preheat oven to 300°F (150°C).

In a large bowl, stir together grapeseed oil, oregano, garlic powder, and sea salt until garlic powder is dissolved and mixture is smooth. Add bread cubes and toss until evenly coated.

Spread bread cubes in a single layer on a baking sheet. Bake, stirring once or twice, until dry, crispy, and golden brown, about 10 to 12 minutes. Let cool on the baking sheet.

....

• Keep in an unsealed container, at room temperature, for up to 1 week.

ALMOND CHILI SAUCE

Full of flavor, with a nice balance between sweet and salty, and with the richness of almond butter. Makes 2 cups (500 mL)

R Raw   **GF** Gluten-Free

Prep Time: 5 minutes • **Special Equipment:** high-speed blender

2 medium cloves garlic, peeled

2 Thai red chilies, chopped

1 tbsp (15 mL) peeled and chopped fresh ginger

¾ cup (175 mL) raw almond butter (page 26)

1½ cups (375 mL) water

½ cup (125 mL) seasoned rice wine vinegar

¼ cup (60 mL) tamari sauce

In a blender, combine all the ingredients. Blend on high speed until creamy.

• Keeps in a sealed container, refrigerated, for up to 1 week.

CUCUMBER AVOCADO DRESSING

A clever and tasty way to pack more vegetables into your salad. Makes 2 cups (500 mL)

R Raw   **GF** Gluten-Free

Prep Time: 5 minutes • **Special Equipment:** high-speed blender

2 medium English cucumbers, peeled and coarsely chopped

1 ripe avocado, peeled and coarsely chopped

2 large handfuls of fresh cilantro leaves

3 medium cloves garlic, peeled

½ cup (125 mL) freshly squeezed lemon juice

6 tbsp (90 mL) grapeseed oil

6 tbsp (90 mL) filtered water

1½ tbsp (22 mL) salt, or to taste

¼ tsp (1 mL) freshly ground black pepper

In a blender, combine all the ingredients. Blend on high speed until smooth and creamy.

• Keeps in a sealed container, refrigerated, for up to 1 week.
• The salt is very important in bringing out all of the other flavors in this light and refreshing dressing, so use a quality salt like Himalayan pink.

GINGER & LEMONGRASS VINAIGRETTE

Clean and fresh-tasting, this is a perfect dressing for summer salads.
Makes 1½ cups (375 mL)

 R Raw   **GF** Gluten-Free   **SND** Super Nutrient-Dense

Prep Time: 5 minutes • **Special Equipment:** high-speed blender, fine-mesh sieve

Handful of fresh cilantro leaves

1½ tbsp (22 mL) coarsely chopped lemongrass

2 tsp (10 mL) agave nectar

½ tsp (2 mL) peeled and coarsely chopped fresh ginger

¾ cup (175 mL) filtered water

½ cup (125 mL) freshly squeezed lime juice

¼ cup (60 mL) grapeseed oil

1 tsp (5 mL) tamari sauce

In a blender, combine all the ingredients. Blend on high speed until emulsified. Strain the dressing through a fine-mesh sieve to remove the lemongrass fibers.

....

• Keeps in a sealed container, refrigerated, for up to 3 weeks.

LEMON VINAIGRETTE

This sweet and punchy dressing is ideal for those transitioning and for those new to salads in general. Makes 1 cup (250 mL)

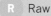 **R** Raw   **GF** Gluten-Free

---

Prep Time: 5 minutes • **Special Equipment:** high-speed blender

½ cup (125 mL) filtered water

¼ cup (60 mL) freshly squeezed lemon juice

2 tsp (10 mL) agave nectar

¼ cup (60 mL) virgin coconut oil, melted

In a blender, combine the water, lemon juice, and agave. While blending on high speed, add the oil in a steady stream. Blend until emulsified.

....

• Keeps in a sealed container, refrigerated, for up to 3 weeks.

RASPBERRY & SWEET BASIL BALSAMIC VINAIGRETTE

Antioxidant-rich, fruity, sweet, and flavorful, here's a dressing perfectly matched to summer salads. Makes 1 cup (250 mL)

R Raw   **GF** Gluten-Free   **SND** Super Nutrient-Dense

Prep Time: 5 minutes • **Special Equipment:** high-speed blender

1 large Medjool date, pitted

4 or 5 fresh sweet basil leaves, torn

¾ cup (175 mL) fresh or frozen raspberries

½ cup (125 mL) filtered water

¼ cup (60 mL) balsamic vinegar

Pinch of freshly ground black pepper

1 tbsp (15 mL) agave nectar or maple syrup

6 tbsp (90 mL) grapeseed oil

In a blender, combine all the ingredients except the grapeseed oil. While blending on high speed, add the oil in a steady stream. Blend until emulsified.

• Keeps in a sealed container, refrigerated, for up to 3 weeks.

SESAME, GINGER & WHITE MISO VINAIGRETTE

A healthier version of an Asian-inspired classic, this vinaigrette goes well on spinach leaves or spring mix greens. Makes 1 cup (250 mL)

R Raw   **GF** Gluten-Free   **SND** Super Nutrient-Dense

Prep Time: 5 minutes • **Special Equipment:** high-speed blender

1 green onion, chopped

1 Medjool date, pitted

3 tbsp (45 mL) white rice miso paste

¾ cup (175 mL) filtered water

½ cup (125 mL) freshly squeezed orange juice

3 tbsp (45 mL) seasoned rice vinegar

1¼ inch (3 cm) knob of ginger

2 tsp (10 mL) toasted sesame oil (optional)

In a blender, combine all the ingredients. Blend on high speed until smooth.

• Keeps in a sealed container, refrigerated, for up to 3 weeks.

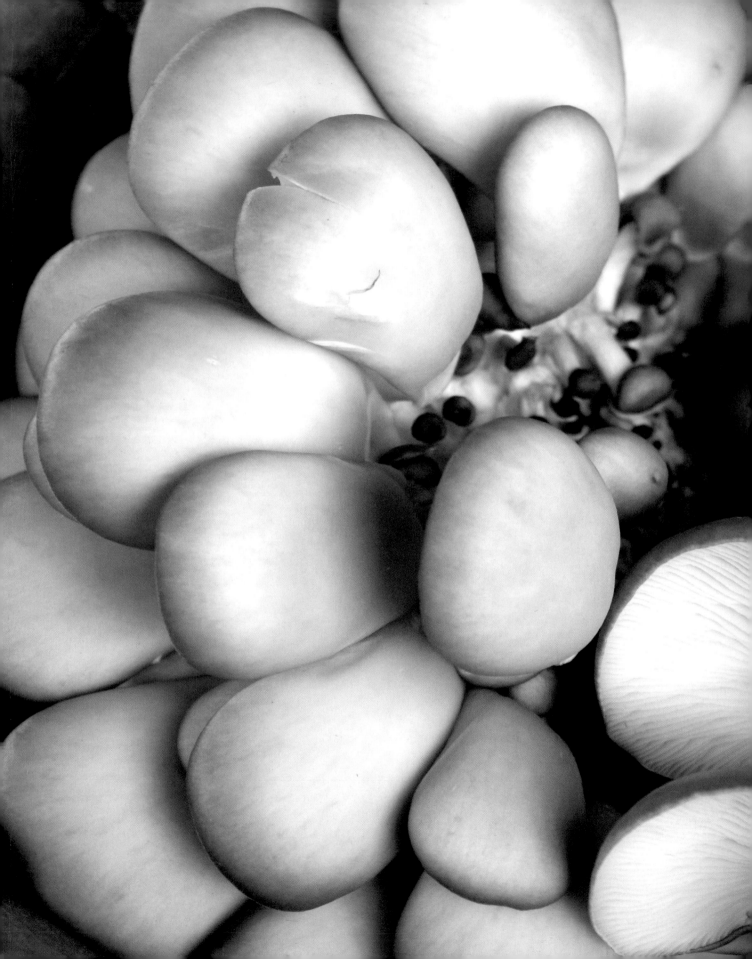

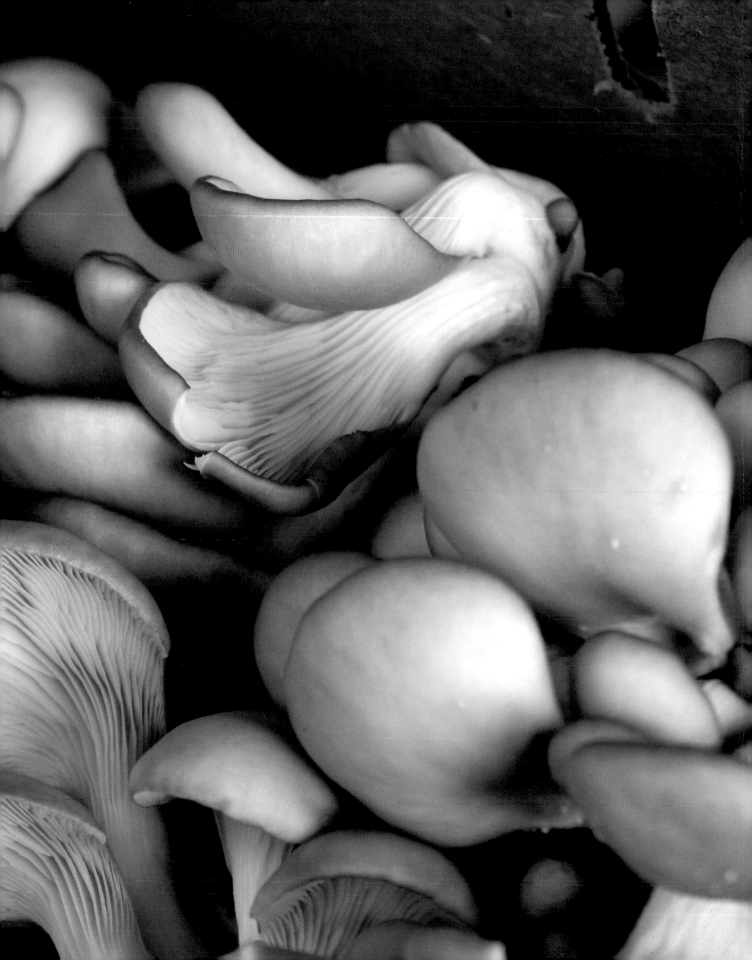

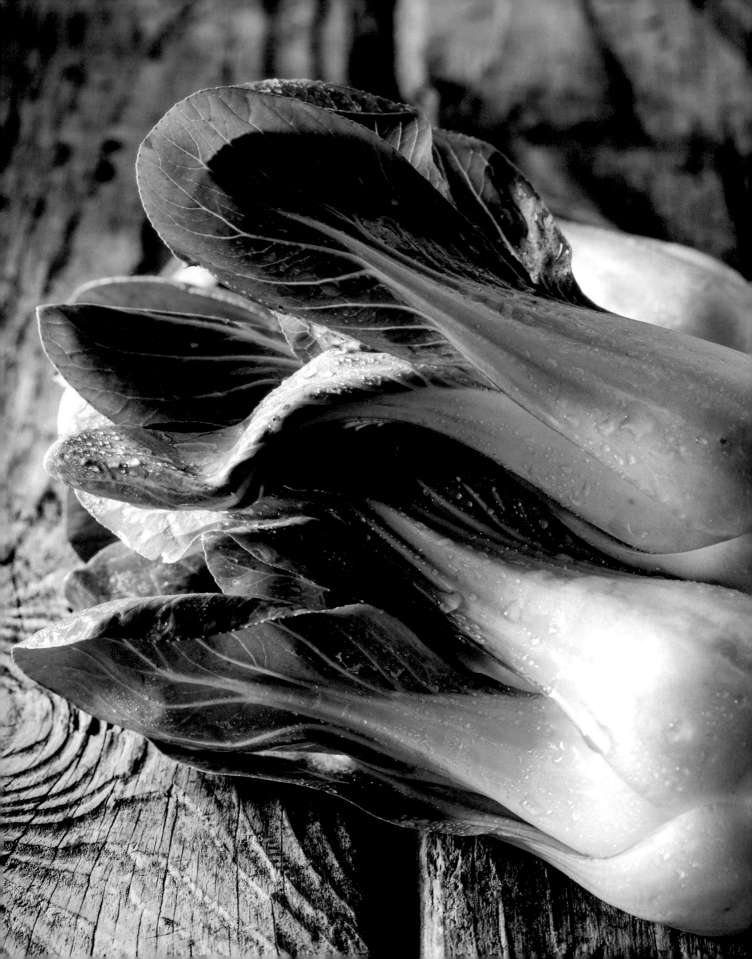

RICE &
NOODLE BOWLS

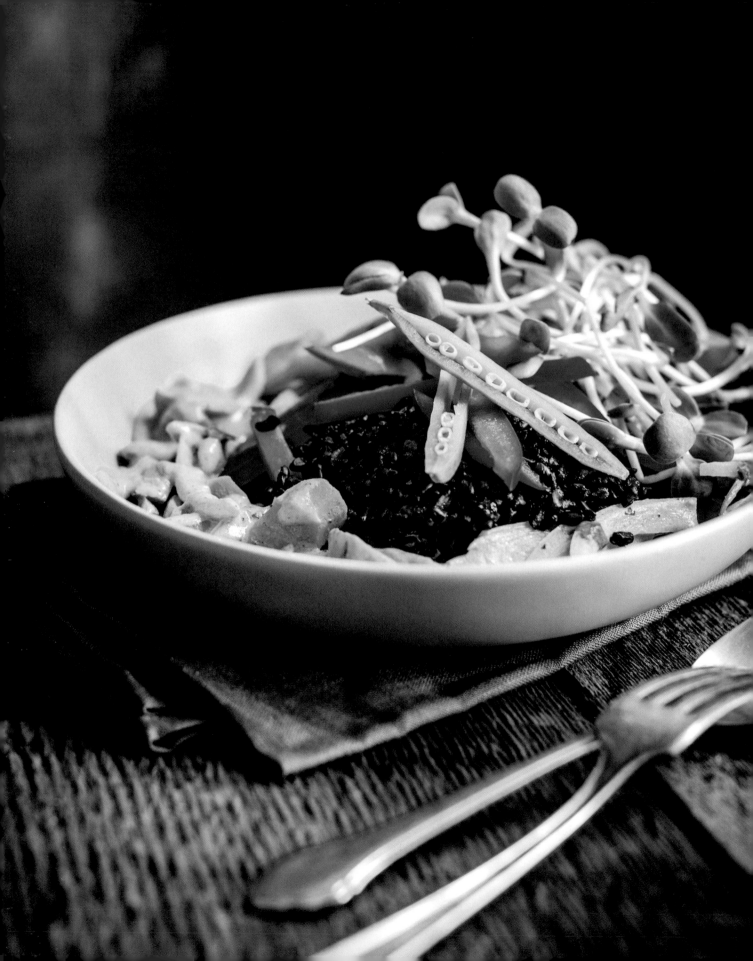

YELLOW PEANUT CURRY RICE BOWL

Loaded with vegetables, this classically flavored, nutrient-packed curry is sure to satisfy. It takes a little time to prepare, but the lively flavors and complementary textures of the vegetables absolutely make it worthwhile. **Serves 4**

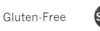 **GF** Gluten-Free **SND** Super Nutrient-Dense

---

Prep Time: 30 to 40 minutes

¼ cup (60 mL) virgin coconut oil

2 cups (500 mL) finely chopped sweet onion

1 cup (250 mL) peeled and diced carrots

1 cup (250 mL) diced celery

2 tbsp (30 mL) pounded and thinly sliced lemongrass

1 tbsp (15 mL) minced garlic

1 tbsp (15 mL) peeled and finely chopped fresh ginger

2 to 3 tbsp (30 to 45 mL) yellow curry paste, or to taste

6 to 8 fresh or frozen lime leaves

1 large sweet red pepper, diced

1 large sweet green pepper, diced

2 cups (500 mL) quartered baby bok choy, washed twice

1½ cups (375 mL) drained canned baby corn

½ cup (125 mL) smooth natural peanut butter

1 cup (250 mL) vegetable stock

4 cans (14 oz/400 mL each) coconut milk, preferably higher in fat

8 to 10 fresh Thai basil leaves, torn

1 cup (250 mL) toasted peanuts, chopped

2 tbsp (30 mL) cane sugar

1 cup (250 mL) whole grain brown rice, cooked

1 cup (250 mL) bean sprouts

4 small handfuls of pea shoots, for garnish

4 small lime wedges, for garnish

In a large pot over medium-high heat, melt the coconut oil. Add the onions, carrots, celery, lemongrass, garlic, and ginger; cook, stirring frequently, for about 5 minutes.

Add the curry paste. Cook, stirring, until the curry paste has melted and mixed with the vegetables, about 5 minutes. Add the lime leaves, red and green peppers, bok choy, and baby corn. Cook for 3 to 4 minutes. Add the peanut butter and cook, stirring, until melted and mixed in.

Reduce heat to medium. Stir in the stock and coconut milk. Add the basil, ½ of the peanuts, and the cane sugar. Bring to a gentle simmer, stirring to blend in the coconut milk, about 15 minutes. Do not let boil or the coconut milk may split.

Serve in large bowls over brown rice with bean sprouts layered on top. Garnish with pea shoots, toasted peanuts, and lime wedges.

THAI GREEN CURRY RICE BOWL

With its distinctive traditional green curry flavor, this fresh-tasting bowl is made up of fiber-rich and nutrient-packed vegetables to keep you satisfied for hours. For a nutritional boost, substitute wild rice for the brown rice. **Serves 4**

 Transition   Gluten-Free **SND** Super Nutrient-Dense

Prep Time: 30 to 40 minutes

2 tbsp (30 mL) virgin coconut oil

2 cups (500 mL) finely chopped sweet onion

2 cups (500 mL) diced celery

3 tbsp (45 mL) pounded and thinly sliced lemongrass

1 tbsp (15 mL) minced garlic

1 tbsp (15 mL) peeled and finely chopped fresh ginger

1½ tsp to 1 tbsp (7 to 15 mL) green curry paste, or to taste

6 to 8 fresh or frozen lime leaves

1 sweet red pepper, diced

2 cups (500 mL) Chinese long beans cut in 2-inch (5 cm) pieces

2 cups (500 mL) snow peas, trimmed

1 cup (250 mL) vegetable stock

8 to 10 fresh Thai basil leaves, torn

8 to 10 fresh mint leaves, torn

4 cans (14 oz/400 mL each) coconut milk, preferably higher in fat

1 cup (250 mL) whole grain brown rice, cooked

1 cup (250 mL) bean sprouts

4 small handfuls of pea shoots, for garnish

2 tbsp (30 mL) sesame seeds, for garnish

4 small lime wedges, for garnish

In a large pot over medium-high heat, melt the coconut oil. Add the onions, celery, lemongrass, garlic, and ginger; cook, stirring frequently, for 5 to 8 minutes.

Add the curry paste. Cook, stirring, until the curry paste has melted and mixed with the vegetables, about 5 minutes. Add the lime leaves, red pepper, long beans, snow peas, and stock. Reduce heat to medium and simmer for 15 minutes.

Add the basil and mint. Stir in the coconut milk. Simmer, stirring occasionally, about 10 minutes. Do not let boil.

Serve in large bowls over brown rice with bean sprouts layered on top. Garnish with pea shoots, sesame seeds, and lime wedges.

THAI RED CURRY RICE BOWL

This vegetable-packed main dish combines several textures with rich complementary flavors. This curry is a Thrive Energy favorite, not only for its terrific flavor but also for its light yet satisfying qualities. Serves 4

 Gluten-Free   **SND** Super Nutrient-Dense

Prep Time: 30 to 40 minutes

½ cup (125 mL) virgin coconut oil

2 cups (500 mL) finely chopped sweet onion

1 cup (250 mL) peeled and diced carrots

1 cup (250 mL) diced celery

2 tbsp (30 mL) pounded and thinly sliced lemongrass

1 tbsp (15 mL) minced garlic

1 tbsp (15 mL) peeled and finely chopped fresh ginger

4 cups (1 L) Asian eggplant cut in ½-inch (1 cm) pieces

1 to 2 tbsp (15 to 30 mL) red curry paste, or to taste

1 sweet red pepper, diced

8 fresh or frozen lime leaves

2 cups (500 mL) canned bamboo shoots, drained

1 cup (250 mL) vegetable stock

8 to 10 fresh Thai basil leaves, torn

2 tbsp (30 mL) cane sugar

4 cans (14 oz/400 mL each) coconut milk, preferably higher in fat

1 cup (250 mL) whole grain brown rice, cooked

1 cup (250 mL) bean sprouts

4 small handfuls of pea shoots, for garnish

2 tbsp (30 mL) sesame seeds, for garnish

4 small lime wedges, for garnish

In a large pot over medium-high heat, melt 2 tbsp (30 mL) of the coconut oil. In a medium pot over medium heat, melt the remaining 6 tbsp (90 mL) coconut oil. In the large pot cook the onions, carrots, celery, lemongrass, garlic, and ginger, stirring frequently, for about 5 minutes.

Meanwhile, in the medium pot, cook the eggplant, stirring gently to coat it with oil, until golden but not fully cooked through, about 10 minutes. Remove with a slotted spoon and drain on several layers of paper towel.

Add the curry paste to the onion mixture. Cook, stirring, until the curry paste has melted and mixed with the vegetables, about 5 minutes. Add the eggplant, red pepper, lime leaves, bamboo shoots, and stock. Reduce heat and simmer for 15 minutes.

Add about three-quarters of the basil and the cane sugar. Stir in the coconut milk. Simmer, stirring occasionally, about 10 minutes. Do not let boil.

Serve in large bowls over brown rice with bean sprouts and the remaining basil layered on top. Garnish with pea shoots, sesame seeds, and lime wedges.

MIDDLE EASTERN RICE BOWL

A main course that will provide sustained energy, this rice bowl is a delicious lunch or dinner option for those with a big appetite. Serves 1

 Gluten-Free

Prep Time: 10 to 15 minutes

Handful of spring mix greens

4 to 6 slices English cucumber (¼-inch/5 mm thick), cut in half

1 tsp (5 mL) extra-virgin olive oil or hemp oil

2 tbsp (30 mL) lemon vinaigrette (page 146)

Sea salt and freshly ground black pepper

1 cup (250 mL) whole grain brown rice, cooked

Small handful of sunflower sprouts

2 large slices tomato

1 large dill pickle, quartered lengthwise

3 falafel patties (page 67), grilled for 4 minutes per side

2 thin red onion rings

Small handful of fresh parsley leaves, torn

¼ cup (60 mL) edamame hummus (page 69)

⅓ to ½ cup (75 to 125 mL) roasted garlic tahini sauce (page 74)

In a medium bowl, combine the spring mix, cucumber, olive oil, 1 tbsp (15 mL) of the vinaigrette, and salt and pepper to taste. Toss gently.

Pile the rice to one side of a large serving bowl. Arrange the salad beside the rice.

Top the salad with the sprouts. Top the rice with the tomatoes, pickles, and falafels. Drizzle the falafels with the remaining vinaigrette and garnish with onion rings and parsley.

Serve with edamame hummus and tahini sauce on the side.

. . . .

• **Use ramekins for the sauces, which makes dipping a lot easier.**

BIG GREEN CURRY KELP NOODLE BOWL

This green curry bowl is made up of fibrous vegetables and mineral-packed kelp noodles. Serves 1 or 2

 GF Gluten-Free   **SND** Super Nutrient-Dense

Prep Time: 10 minutes

Special Equipment: high-speed juicer, blender, mandoline with julienne blade or julienne peeler

Curry Sauce

½ ripe avocado, peeled

1 tsp (5 mL) chopped lemongrass

½ tsp (2 mL) peeled and chopped fresh ginger

½ tsp (2 mL) green curry paste or to taste

2 cups (500 mL) coconut milk

¼ cup (60 mL) freshly squeezed carrot juice

Sea salt and freshly ground black pepper, to taste

Noodle Bowl

1 cup (250 mL) Asian julienned vegetable mix (page 128)

½ cup (125 mL) bean sprouts

1 tbsp (15 mL) freshly squeezed lime juice

1 tsp (5 mL) sesame oil

Small handful of fresh cilantro leaves, torn

Handful of fresh Thai basil leaves, torn

1 cup (250 mL) packed raw kelp noodles, rinsed

⅓ cup (75 mL) peeled and julienned watermelon radish, for garnish

½ avocado, sliced thinly

¼ cup (60 mL) raw cashews

1 tsp (5 mL) sesame seeds, for garnish

For the curry sauce, in a blender, combine all the ingredients. Blend on high speed until creamy and smooth. Set aside.

For the noodle bowl, in a medium bowl, combine the Asian vegetable mix, bean sprouts, lime juice, sesame oil, cilantro, and most of the basil. Toss well.

Place the kelp noodles in a large serving bowl. Top with the vegetable mixture, trying to gain as much height as possible. Pour the curry sauce down the side of the bowl, being careful not to disturb the noodles and vegetables too much, until the noodles and some of the vegetables are immersed. You may not need all the sauce. Garnish with the watermelon radish, sliced avocado, cashews, sesame seeds, and the remaining basil.

PAD THAI RICE NOODLE BOWL

This pad Thai recipe is loaded with inflammation-reducing ingredients combined to bring out diverse flavors and textures. Kelp noodles pack even more minerals into your meal, while providing some extra crunch as well. Serves 1

R Raw   **T** Transition

Prep Time: 12 minutes
Special Equipment: mandoline with julienne blade or julienne peeler

1 cup (250 mL) medium rice noodles, cooked for about 6 minutes, drained and cooled, or raw kelp noodles, rinsed

1 cup (250 mL) Asian julienned vegetable mix (page 128)

4 to 6 tbsp (60 to 90 mL) pad Thai sauce (page 76), or more to taste

2 tbsp (30 mL) ginger & lemongrass vinaigrette (page 146)

2 tbsp (30 mL) almond chili sauce (page 145)

¼ cup (60 mL) bean sprouts

6 to 8 snow peas, trimmed and thinly sliced lengthwise

½ medium watermelon radish, peeled and julienned

3 tbsp (45 mL) toasted peanuts (or 10 to 12 cashews), chopped

6 or 7 fresh Thai basil leaves, torn

4 or 5 fresh mint leaves, torn

3 slices tempeh, grilled on each side for 2 to 3 minutes (transition option)

½ ripe avocado, peeled, thinly sliced

A handful of pea shoots, for garnish

2 lime wedges, for garnish

1 tsp (5 mL) sesame oil

In a medium bowl, combine the noodles, Asian vegetable mix, pad Thai sauce, and 1 tbsp (15 mL) of the vinaigrette. Toss gently until everything is lightly coated with sauce.

Transfer the noodle mixture to a large serving bowl. Drizzle with almond chili sauce. Letting the ingredients fall in place naturally, and trying to gain height, top with the bean sprouts, snow peas, and radish. Sprinkle with the peanuts, basil, and mint.

Stack the tempeh slices (if using) and slice diagonally. Place the tempeh and fan out the avocado to one side of the noodles. Garnish with pea shoots and lime wedges. Drizzle with the remainder of the ginger & lemongrass vinaigrette and sesame oil.

· ·

• For a raw version, leave out the tempeh and peanuts. Use the raw kelp noodles instead of cooked rice noodles.
• Make sure you use enough pad Thai sauce, or else the water released from the Asian julienned vegetables when you chew them will dilute the flavors.

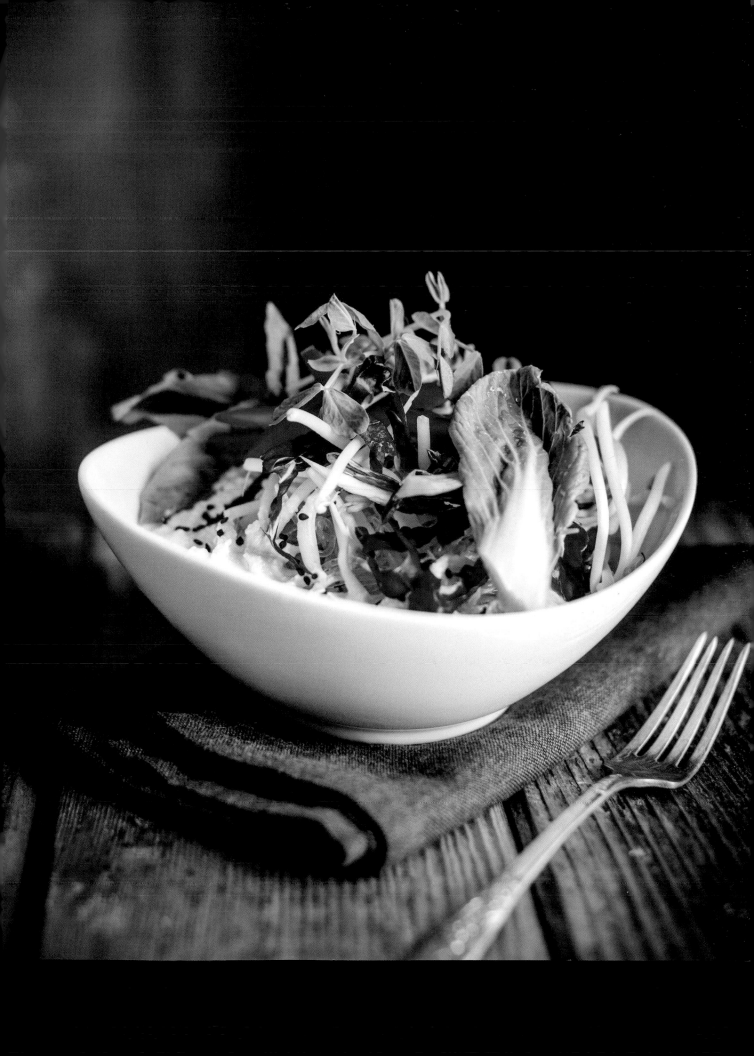

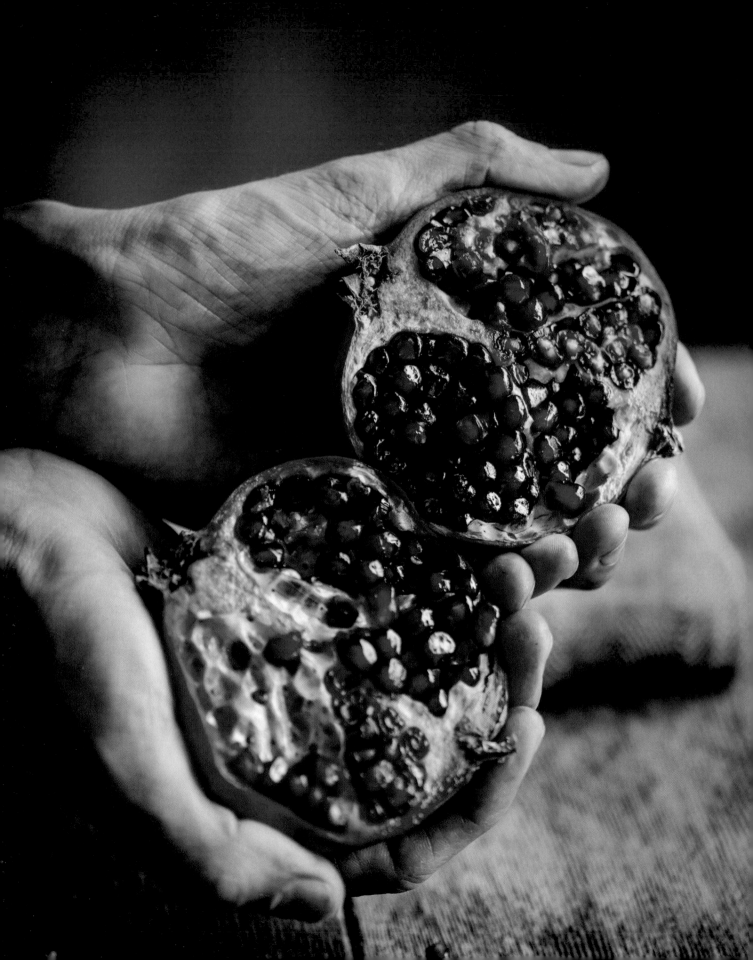

SMOOTHIES, FRESH JUICES & WARM DRINKS

COCONUT-LIME BLISS

This rich, decadent smoothie is packed with goodness, making it ideal for those transitioning to a clean, whole foods, plant-based diet, and for athletes who work out for an hour or more a day. Serves 1/Makes 2¼ cups (550 mL)

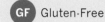 **T** Transition   **GF** Gluten-Free

Prep Time: 2 to 3 minutes • **Equipment:** high-speed blender

2 fresh or frozen lime leaves

Zest of ½ lime

¾ cup (175 mL) coconut water

2 tbsp (30 mL) unsweetened shredded coconut

2 tbsp (30 mL) coconut milk

1 tbsp (15 mL) chopped lemongrass

1 scoop Coconut Bliss gelato (transition option)

1 tsp (5 mL) agave or coconut nectar (if not using Coconut Bliss gelato)

About 2 cups (500 mL) ice cubes

In a blender, combine all the ingredients except the ice. Add ice to about 1 inch (2.5 cm) above the liquid line. Blend on high speed until smooth and creamy.

LEMON-GINGER ZINGER

With anti-inflammation and alkalizing properties, this drink is as functional as it is delicious. This is a crushed ice/smoothie blend and is slightly thinner in consistency than most smoothies. Serves 1/Makes 2¼ cups (550 mL)

R Raw   **GF** Gluten-Free

Prep Time: 3 to 4 minutes • **Equipment:** high-speed blender

3 or 4 fresh sweet basil leaves

1-inch (2.5 cm) knob of fresh ginger, peeled

½ cup (125 mL) coconut water

¼ cup (60 mL) freshly squeezed lemon juice

2 tbsp (30 mL) agave or coconut nectar (optional)

1 tbsp (15 mL) pure vanilla extract

About 3 cups (750 mL) ice cubes

In a blender, combine all the ingredients except the ice. Add ice to about 2 inches (5 cm) above the liquid line. Blend on high speed until smooth.

TROPICAL BREEZE

Tropical flavors with the refreshing taste of lemongrass. Serves 1/Makes 2¼ cups (550 mL)

GF Gluten-Free

Prep Time: 3 to 4 minutes • **Equipment:** high-speed blender

1 cup (250 mL) chopped pineapple

Zest of ½ lime

1 tbsp (15 mL) chopped lemongrass

1 tbsp (15 mL) agave nectar

2 tbsp (30 mL) unsweetened shredded coconut or 1 tbsp (15 mL) coconut butter

2 tbsp (30 mL) coconut milk

¾ cup (175 mL) coconut water

About 2 cups (500 mL) ice cubes

In a blender, combine all the ingredients except the ice. Add ice to about 1 inch (2.5 cm) above the liquid line. Blend on high speed until smooth and creamy.

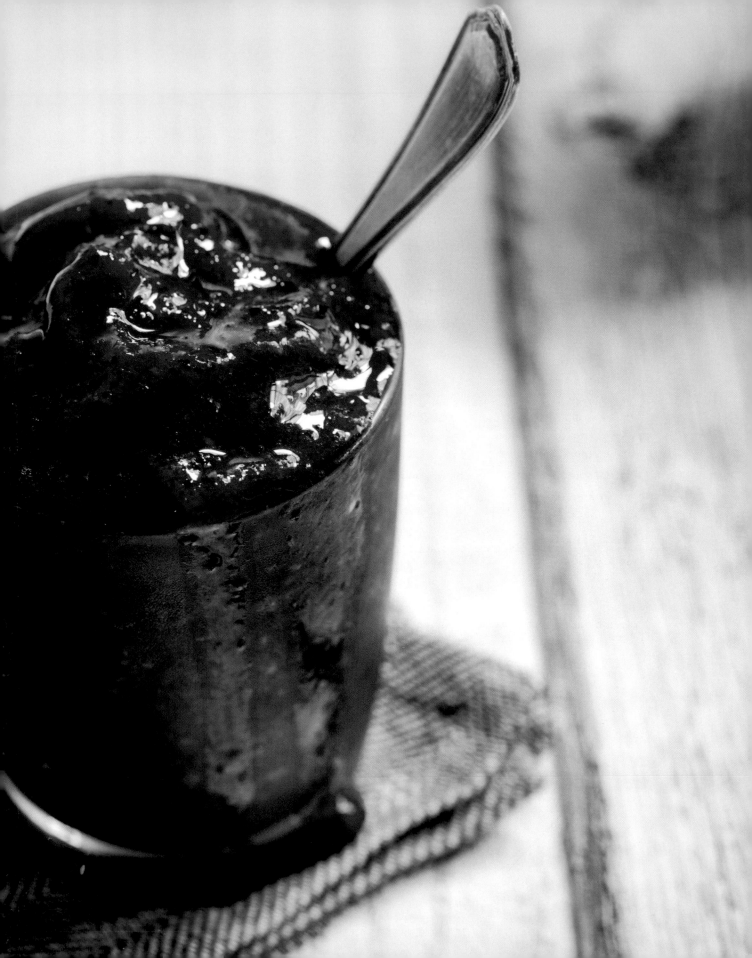

SUPER-FRUIT SANGRIA

Even people who say they don't like "healthy drinks" will love this. The properly balanced and complementary flavors of the fruit make it delicious.

Serves 1/Makes 2¼ cups (550 mL)

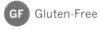 Gluten-Free   **SND** Super Nutrient-Dense

---

Prep Time: 5 minutes • **Special Equipment:** high-speed blender

4 or 5 fresh or frozen strawberries

10 fresh or frozen raspberries

½ cup (125 mL) fresh or frozen blueberries

⅓ cup (75 mL) chopped pineapple

2 fresh mint leaves

Zest of ½ orange

Zest of ½ lemon

Zest of ½ lime

2 tbsp (30 mL) freshly squeezed orange juice

2 tbsp (30 mL) freshly squeezed lemon juice

2 tbsp (30 mL) freshly squeezed lime juice

2 tbsp (30 mL) pomegranate juice

2 tbsp (30 mL) acai berry juice

6 tbsp (90 mL) coconut water

2 tbsp (30 mL) agave nectar or maple syrup

1 tbsp (15 mL) pure vanilla extract

About 2 cups (500 mL) ice cubes

In a blender, combine all the ingredients except the ice. Add ice to about 1 inch (2.5 cm) above the liquid line. Blend on high speed until smooth and creamy.

. . . .

• If using frozen fruit, use less ice.

STRAWBERRY-KIWI-PEACH PLEASER

This smoothie is fantastic when made with fresh fruit in season, but it's also delicious year-round with frozen fruit. Include the optional sweetener if you've done a workout earlier in the day or will later in the day, but leave it out if you're not performing physical activity that day. Serves 1/Makes 2¼ cups (550 mL)

R Raw   **GF** Gluten-Free

Prep Time: 2 to 3 minutes • **Equipment:** high-speed blender

1 cup (250 mL) fresh or frozen strawberries

1 cup (250 mL) peeled and chopped kiwifruit

1 cup (250 mL) chopped or sliced fresh or frozen peaches (about 1 large peach)

¾ cup (175 mL) coconut water

4 tsp (20 mL) agave nectar or maple syrup (optional)

About 2 cups (500 mL) ice cubes

In a blender, combine all the ingredients except the ice. Add ice to about 1 inch (2.5 cm) above the liquid line. Blend on high speed until smooth.

....

• If using frozen fruit, use less ice.

COCONUT-CASHEW-DATE ENERGY BOOST

Sustained energy in a decadent form, this smoothie is ideal for days when you are really active or working out. It's packed with clean-burning carbohydrates, high-quality fats, electrolyte-rich coconut water, and energy-boosting healthy medium-chain triglyceride fats. Serves 1/Makes 2¼ cups (550 mL)

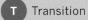 **T** Transition   **GF** Gluten-Free

---

Prep Time: 3 to 4 minutes • **Equipment:** high-speed blender

In a blender, combine all the ingredients except the ice. Add ice to about 1 inch (2.5 cm) above the liquid line. Blend on high speed until smooth and creamy.

....

• Using frozen banana gives this drink a creamy texture. If using frozen fruit, use less ice.

½ fresh or frozen banana

6 cashews

1 tbsp (15 mL) raw cashew butter

1 tbsp (15 mL) dried unsweetened coconut

1 tbsp (15 mL) chopped pitted Medjool date

1 tsp (5 mL) chopped lemongrass

¼ cup (60 mL) or 1 scoop Coconut Bliss gelato (optional, but highly recommended on long workout days)

½ cup (125 mL) unsweetened almond milk (or homemade, page 23)

½ cup (125 mL) coconut water

1 tsp (5 mL) pure vanilla extract

About 2 cups (500 mL) ice cubes

MANGO-ORANGE CRUSH

Rich and creamy, this classic smoothie is a summertime favorite. With the addition of the Big Orange Smoothie Powder Mix, this smoothie is loaded with immune-boosting properties. Serves 1/Makes 2¼ cups (550 mL)

 Raw   **GF** Gluten-Free   **SND** Super Nutrient-Dense

Prep Time: 2 to 3 minutes • **Special Equipment:** high-speed blender

1 Medjool date, pitted

1 cup (250 mL) peeled and chopped fresh or frozen mango

6 tbsp (90 mL) freshly squeezed orange juice

6 tbsp (90 mL) pure mango juice

⅓ cup (75 mL) unsweetened shredded coconut

¼ cup (60 mL) coconut water

½ tsp (2 mL) big orange smoothie powder mix (page 216)

About 2 cups (500 mL) ice cubes

In a blender, combine all the ingredients except the ice. Add ice to about 1 inch (2.5 cm) above the liquid line. Blend on high speed until smooth.

···

• If using frozen fruit, use less ice.

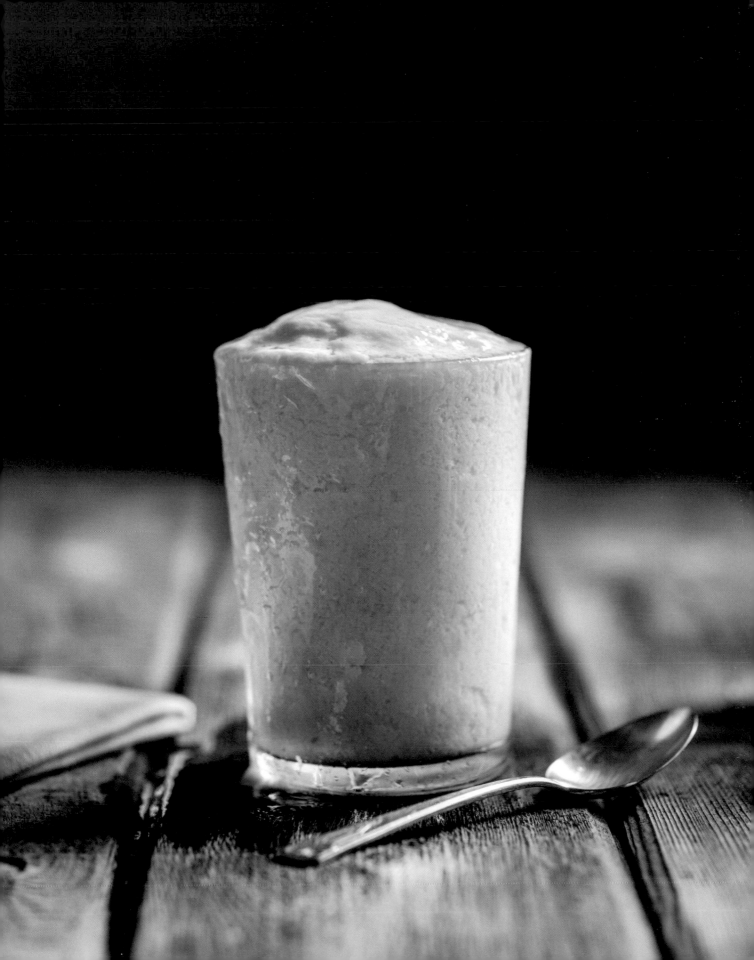

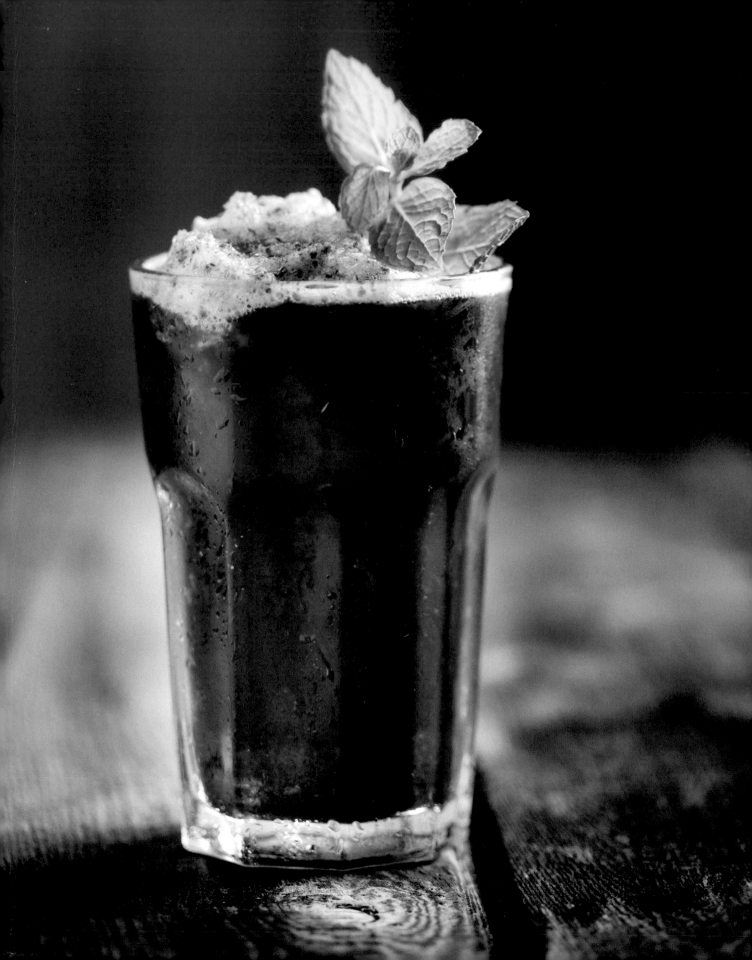

KALE MOJITO

Rich in chlorophyll, kale is one of the healthiest vegetables. It's right at home in this refreshing Thrive Energy super-power smoothie. Serves 1/Makes 2¼ cups (550 mL)

R Raw   **GF** Gluten-Free   **SND** Super Nutrient-Dense

Prep Time: 3 to 4 minutes • **Special Equipment:** high-speed blender

In a blender, combine all the ingredients except the ice. Add ice to about 2 inches (5 cm) above the liquid line. Blend on high speed until smooth. Some small pieces of kale and mint will remain.

2 medium kale leaves, stems removed

Handful of fresh mint leaves

Zest of ½ lime

3 tbsp (45 mL) freshly squeezed lime juice

⅔ cup (150 mL) coconut water

2 tbsp (30 mL) coconut nectar

About 3 cups (750 mL) ice cubes

SUPER-BERRY FRENZY

This antioxidant-rich smoothie is ideal for those who are active. It's perfect right after a workout to help combat free radical damage done by the increased oxygen uptake during exercise. Serves 1/Makes 2¼ cups (550 mL)

 R Raw   **GF** Gluten-Free   **SND** Super Nutrient-Dense

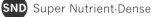

Prep Time: 2 to 3 minutes • **Special Equipment:** high-speed blender

1 Medjool date, pitted

8 fresh or frozen raspberries

8 fresh or frozen cranberries

4 fresh or frozen strawberries

¼ cup (60 mL) fresh or frozen blueberries

1 tbsp (15 mL) goji berries

½ tsp (2 mL) noni powder (or torn-up nori sheets)

½ cup (125 mL) coconut water

¼ cup (60 mL) acai berry juice

¼ cup (60 mL) pure blueberry juice

1 tbsp (15 mL) pure vanilla extract

About 2 cups (500 mL) ice cubes

In a blender, combine all the ingredients except the ice. Add ice to about 1 inch (2.5 cm) above the liquid line. Blend on high speed until smooth.

• If using frozen fruit, use less ice.
• To make this drink even more nutritious, replace the goji berries with 1 serving of berry-flavor Vega One Nutritional Shake.

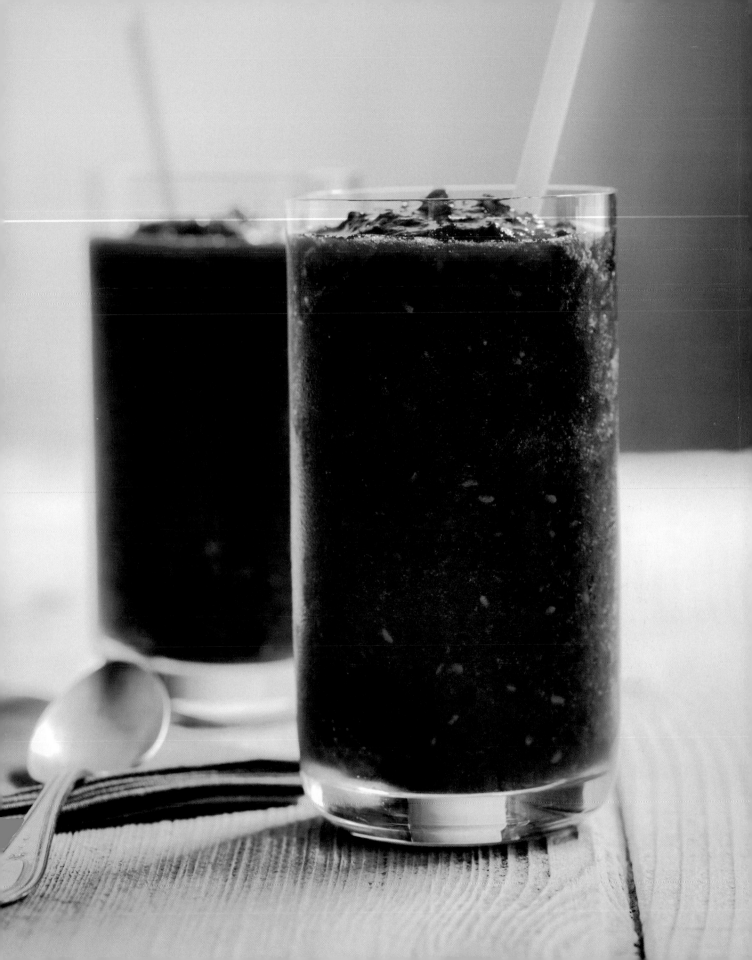

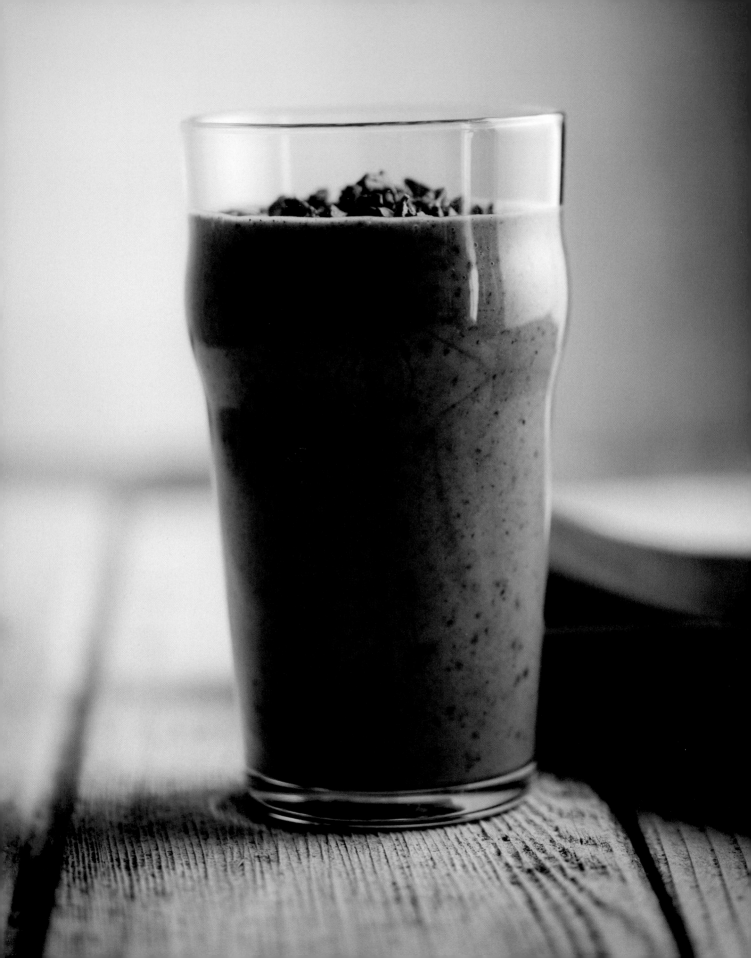

CHOCOLATE-ALMOND DECADENCE

This is not your normal smoothie. It is one of the richest, most decadent creations in this cookbook. An instant classic, this Thrive Energy smoothie has helped transition many a standard-American-diet eater into a plant-based whole food advocate. Serves 1/Makes 2¼ cups (550 mL)

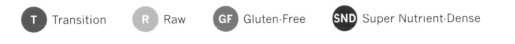

T Transition   **R** Raw   **GF** Gluten-Free   **SND** Super Nutrient-Dense

---

Prep Time: 2 to 3 minutes • **Special Equipment:** high-speed blender

In a blender, combine all the ingredients except the ice and cacao nibs. Add ice to about 1 inch (2.5 cm) above the liquid line. Blend on high speed until smooth. Serve topped with cacao nibs.

. . . .

- If using frozen fruit, use less ice.
- If you prefer a thicker, creamier smoothie, add ¼ peeled ripe avocado.
- To boost this smoothie's nutritional value, replace the cacao powder and chocolate powder mix with 1 scoop of chocolate-flavor Vega One Nutritional Shake.

1 Medjool date, pitted

1 tbsp (15 mL) cacao powder

1 tbsp (15 mL) goji berries

1 tbsp (15 mL) vanilla bean powder or extract

1 tbsp (15 mL) almond butter (page 26)

¼ avocado (optional, for extra creaminess and EFA)

1 tsp (5 mL) super chocolate powder mix (page 217)

½ cup (125 mL) coconut water

½ cup (125 mL) unsweetened almond milk (or homemade, page 23)

1 tbsp (15 mL) coconut nectar

About 2 cups (500 mL) ice cubes

1 tbsp (15 mL) cacao nibs

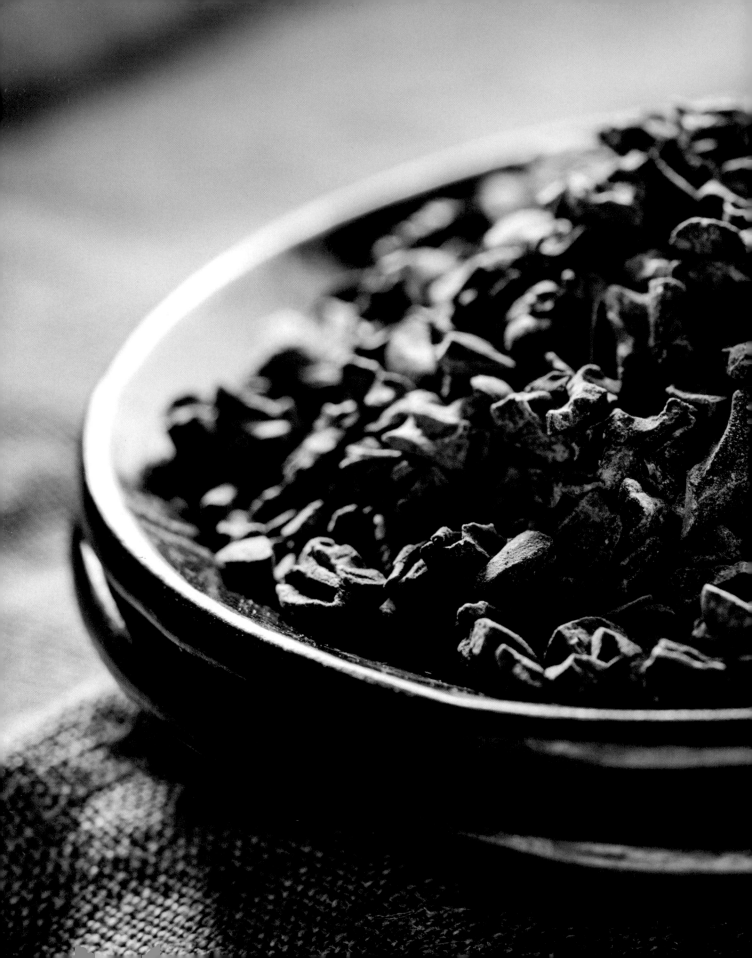

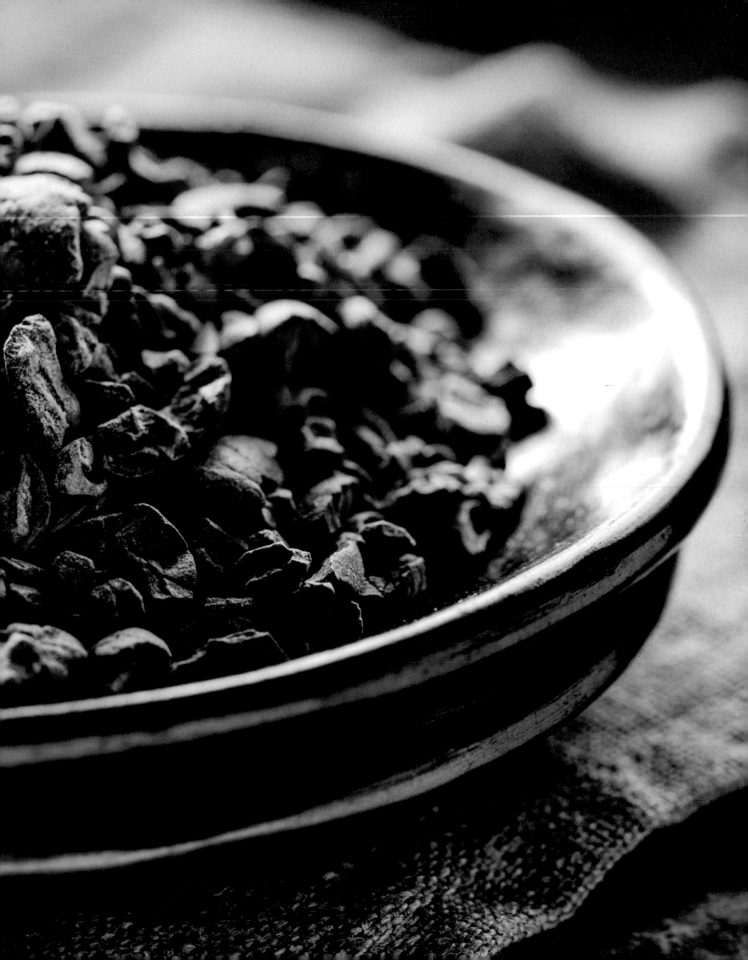

CREAMY CHOCOLATE-AVOCADO DELIGHT

Rich, creamy, and filling, this premium Thrive Energy smoothie will keep kids and adults alike going for hours. Serves 1/Makes 2¼ cups (550 mL)

T Transition   **R** Raw   **GF** Gluten-Free

Prep Time: 3 to 4 minutes • **Special Equipment:** high-speed blender

2 large Medjool dates, pitted

½ ripe avocado, peeled

1 tbsp (15 mL) vegan dark chocolate chips

1 tbsp (15 mL) cacao nibs

1 tbsp (15 mL) cacao powder

1 tbsp (15 mL) raw cashew butter

½ cup (125 mL) chocolate almond milk (or homemade, page 23)

½ cup (125 mL) coconut water

About 2 cups (500 mL) ice cubes

In a blender, combine all the ingredients except the ice. Add ice to about 1 inch (2.5 cm) above the liquid line. Blend on high speed until smooth and creamy.

CHOCOLATE-PEPPERMINT MATCHA MAGIC

Creamy, chocolate peppermint with the kick of phytochemical-rich matcha green tea. A satisfying, energy-sustaining coffee substitute. Serves 1/Makes 2¼ cups (550 mL)

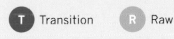 **T** Transition   **R** Raw   **GF** Gluten-Free

---

Prep Time: 3 to 4 minutes • **Special Equipment:** high-speed blender

In a blender, combine all the ingredients except the ice. Add ice to about 1 inch (2.5 cm) above the liquid line. Blend on high speed until smooth and creamy.

2 large Medjool dates, pitted

½ avocado, peeled

4 or 5 fresh mint leaves

1 tbsp (15 mL) cacao nibs

1 tbsp (15 mL) vegan dark chocolate chips

½ tbsp (7 mL) matcha green tea powder

6 or 7 drops pure mint extract

½ cup (125 mL) unsweetened almond milk (or homemade, page 23)

½ cup (125 mL) coconut water

1 tbsp (15 mL) cacao powder

About 2 cups (500 mL) ice cubes

HEAVENLY PISTACHIO BLISS

Truly a full-flavored, creamy smoothie that contains high-quality fats. Drizzling it with lacuma caramel sauce will boost its nutritional content as well as give it a delicious dessert quality. Serves 1/Makes 2¼ cups (550 mL)

T Transition　　**R** Raw　　**GF** Gluten-Free

Prep Time: 3 to 4 minutes • Equipment: high-speed blender

¼ avocado, peeled

½ cup (125 mL) unsalted pistachios

2 tbsp (30 mL) cacao nibs

1 tbsp (15 mL) chopped pitted Medjool date

1 tsp (5 mL) pure vanilla extract

7 oz (200 mL) unsweetened almond milk (or homemade, page 23)

1 tbsp (15 mL) agave nectar

Pinch of sea salt

About 2 cups (500 mL) ice cubes

1 tbsp (15 mL) lacuma caramel sauce (page 214)

In a blender, combine all the ingredients except the ice and caramel sauce. Add ice to about 1 inch (2.5 cm) above the liquid line. Blend on high speed until smooth and creamy. Serve drizzled with caramel sauce, if using.

VANILLA-ALMOND-MOCHA MOTIVATOR

A decadent endurance energy-booster that is made up of fats, cacao, and coffee beans. This is the smoothie to keep you going if you are active, and it's a Thrive Energy pre-bike ride favorite. Serves 1/Makes 2¼ cups (550 mL)

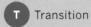 **T** Transition   **GF** Gluten-Free

---

Prep Time: 3 to 4 minutes • Equipment: high-speed blender, espresso maker

In a blender, combine all the ingredients except the ice. Add ice to about 1 inch (2.5 cm) above the liquid line. Blend on high speed until smooth and creamy.

....

• Use decaffeinated coffee beans for a low-caffeine alternative.

2 large Medjool dates, pitted

4 coffee beans (or ½-oz/15 mL espresso shot)

1 tbsp (15 mL) cacao nibs

1 tbsp (15 mL) vegan dark chocolate chips

1 tbsp (15 mL) vanilla powder or extract

1 tbsp (15 mL) almond butter (page 26)

1 tsp (5 mL) cacao butter

¾ cup (175 mL) unsweetened almond milk (or homemade, page 23)

¼ cup (60 mL) coconut water

About 2 cups (500 mL) ice cubes

THAI AVOCADO REFRESHER

A classic clean, simple, and fresh-tasting smoothie that's ideal as an energy-sustaining mid-afternoon snack. Serves 1/Makes 2¼ cups (550 mL)

R Raw   **GF** Gluten-Free

Prep Time: 3 to 4 minutes • **Special Equipment:** high-speed blender

½ avocado, peeled

2 large Medjool dates, pitted

1 tbsp (15 mL) chopped lemongrass

1 tbsp (15 mL) pure vanilla extract

½ cup (125 mL) unsweetened almond milk (or homemade, page 23)

½ cup (125 mL) coconut water

About 2 cups (500 mL) ice cubes

In a blender, combine all the ingredients except the ice. Add ice to about 1 inch (2.5 cm) above the liquid line. Blend until smooth and creamy.

....

• Use the remaining lemongrass stem as garnish, if you like. It adds a little more flavor and a fresh smell.

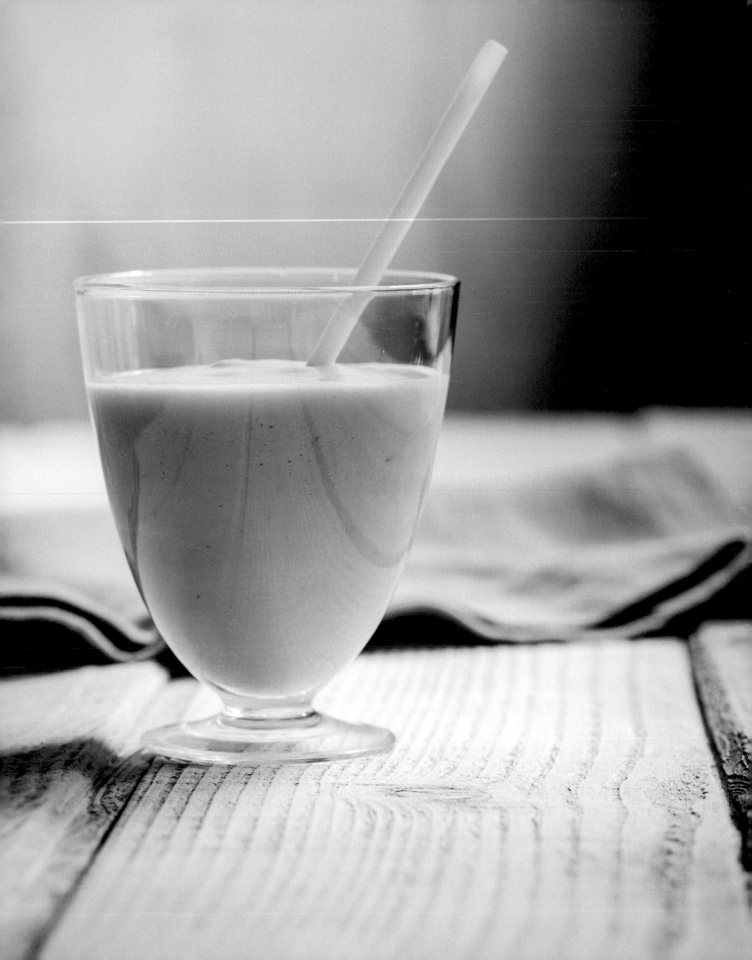

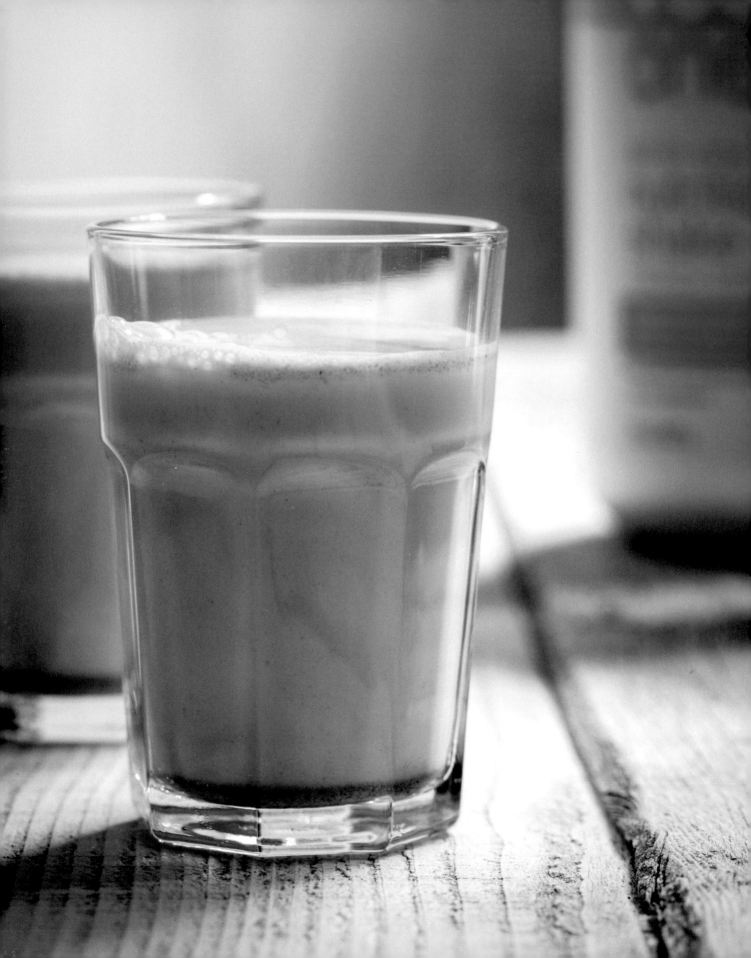

BREAKFAST ENERGIZER

Chock-full of nutrition, this smoothie will have you going strong all morning. It contains slow-burning carbohydrates, essential fatty acids, and high-quality, alkaline-forming protein. Unlike traditional breakfasts, this one digests easily. As a result, not as much blood will be drawn to the stomach, leaving more to circulate through the brain, enhancing the ability to think clearly and work efficiently. You can skip the Vega EFA Oil Blend if you have a high-quality EFA on your salad later in the day. Serves 1/Makes 2¼ cups (550 mL)

 Transition   Gluten-Free   Super Nutrient-Dense

Prep Time: 2 to 3 minutes • **Equipment:** high-speed blender

In a blender, combine all the ingredients except the ice. Add ice to about 1 inch (2.5 cm) above the liquid line. Blend on high speed until smooth and creamy.

. . . .

• If using frozen fruit, use less ice.

1 large or 2 small Medjool dates, pitted and chopped

½ large or 1 small fresh or frozen banana

½ cup (125 mL) fresh or frozen blueberries

¼ cup (60 mL) gluten-free rolled oats

1 tbsp (15 mL) almond butter (page 26)

1 tsp (5 mL) chia seeds

1 scoop French vanilla–flavor Vega One Nutritional Shake

½ cup (125 mL) coconut water or wild blueberry juice

½ cup (125 mL) unsweetened almond milk (or homemade, page 23)

1 tbsp (15 mL) Vega EFA Oil Blend (optional)

About 2 cups (500 mL) ice cubes

BIG GREEN ENERGY CHARGER

This alkaline-forming, anti-inflammation smoothie is full of nutrients and a Thrive Energy breakfast staple. **Serves 1/Makes 2¼ cups (550 mL)**

T Transition   **GF** Gluten-Free   **SND** Super Nutrient-Dense

---

Prep Time: 5 to 6 minutes
Special Equipment: slow speed juice extractor, high-speed blender

½ avocado, peeled

3 medium kale leaves, stems removed

Handful of spinach

2 Medjool dates, pitted

½ scoop French vanilla–flavor Vega One Nutritional Shake

1 cup (250 mL) coconut water

1 tbsp (15 mL) freshly squeezed wheatgrass juice

1 tbsp (15 mL) pure vanilla extract or powder

¼ tsp (1 mL) chlorella powder

About 2 cups (500 mL) ice cubes

In a blender, combine all the ingredients except the ice. Add ice to about 1 inch (2.5 cm) above the liquid line. Blend on high speed until smooth and creamy.

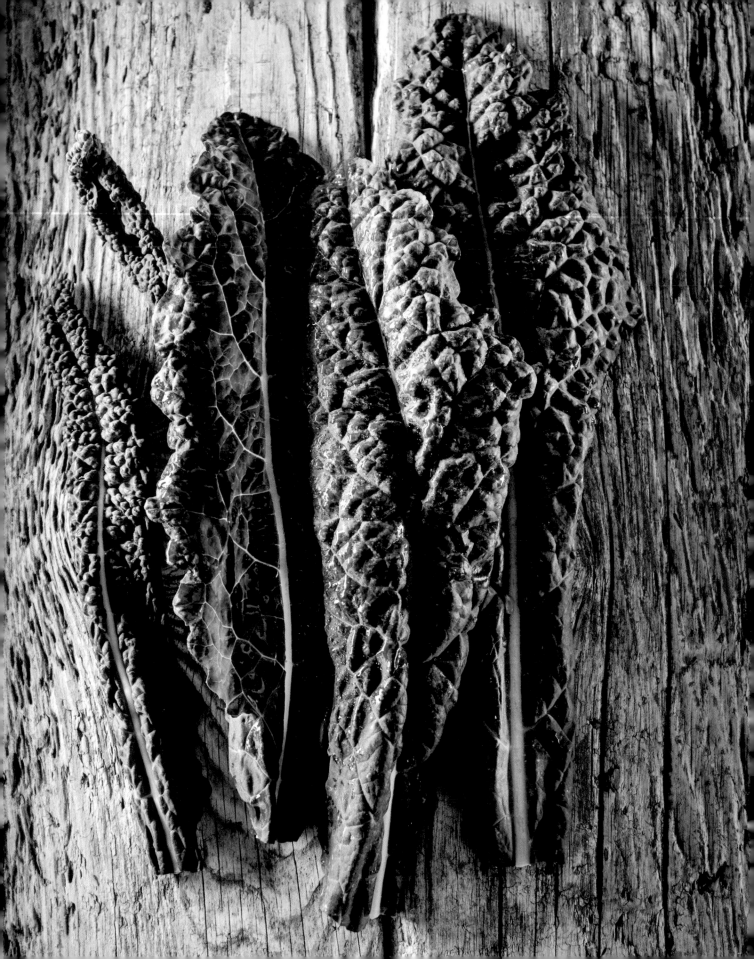

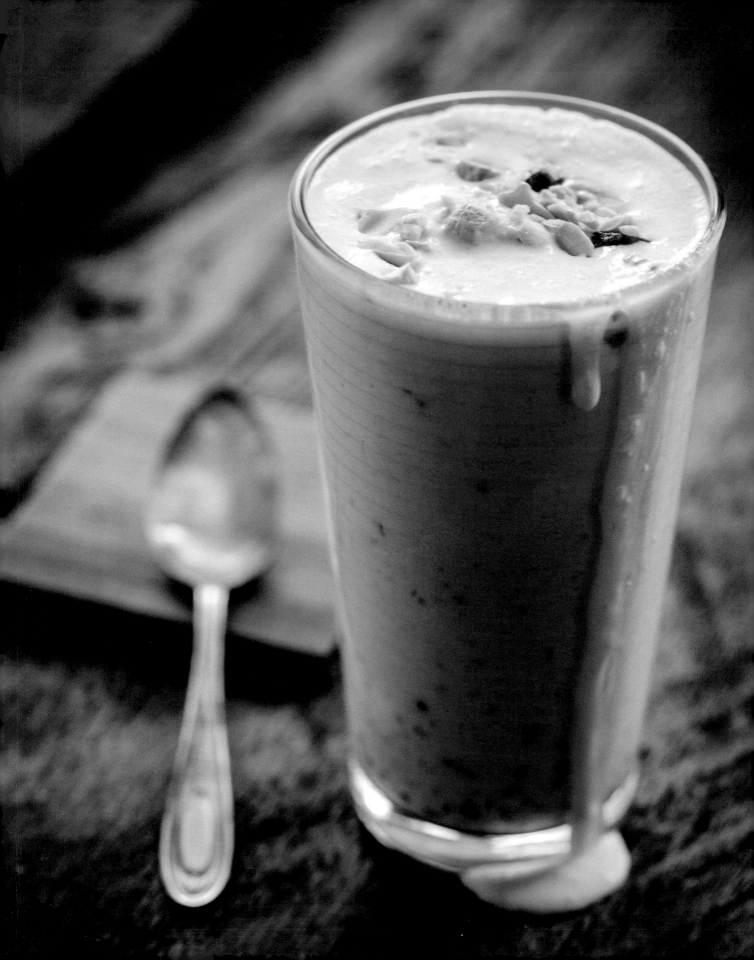

CHOCOLATE CHIP FRENCH VANILLA SMOOTHIE

Possibly the most delicious and satisfying Thrive Energy smoothie, this is a go-to choice for those who love the combination of vanilla and chocolate. Serves 1/Makes 2¼ cups (550 mL)

 Transition   GF Gluten-Free

Prep Time: 2 to 3 minutes • **Special Equipment:** high-speed blender

In a blender, combine all the ingredients except the ice. Add ice to about 1 inch (2.5 cm) above the liquid line. Blend on high speed until smooth.

1 Medjool date, pitted

1 tbsp (15 mL) chia seeds

1 tbsp (15 mL) almond butter (page 26)

1 tbsp (15 mL) cacao nibs

1 tbsp (15 mL) vegan dark chocolate chips

1 scoop French vanilla–flavor Vega One Nutritional Shake

6 tbsp (90 mL) unsweetened almond milk (or homemade, page 23)

6 tbsp (90 mL) coconut water

1½ tsp (7 mL) pure vanilla extract or powder

About 2 cups (500 mL) ice cubes

MIGHTY KING CHLOROPHYLL

A Thrive Energy staple juice, this chlorophyll-packed, mineral-rich, phytochemical-heavy, alkalizing elixir will energize you with a small amount of natural sugar from the apple and pear. Serves 1/Makes 2¼ cups (550 mL)

 R Raw   **GF** Gluten-Free   **SND** Super Nutrient-Dense

Prep Time: 4 to 5 minutes
Special Equipment: slow-speed juice extractor, high-speed juicer

2 large kale leaves, stems removed

Handful of spinach

¼ English cucumber (unpeeled)

1 large celery rib, trimmed

1 large apple (unpeeled)

1 pear

¼ tsp (1 mL) chlorella powder (optional)

1 tbsp (15 mL) wheatgrass juice (optional)

1 tbsp (15 mL) freshly squeezed lemon juice

Juice the kale and spinach in a slow-speed juice extractor. Juice the cucumber, celery, apple, and pear in a high-speed juicer.

Stir together the two juices and the chlorella powder (if using), making sure there are no lumps. Stir in the wheatgrass juice (if using) and lemon juice.

....

• Wheatgrass and chlorella are both chlorophyll-rich and will therefore help reduce inflammation. The lemon juice not only smooths out the flavors but also helps with chlorophyll absorption.

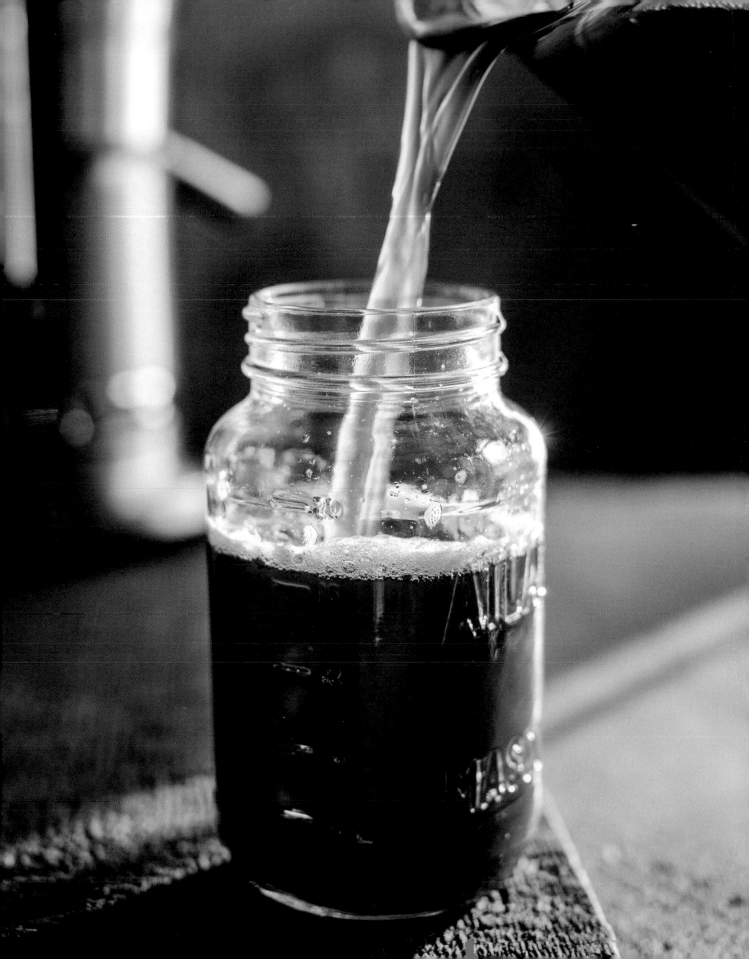

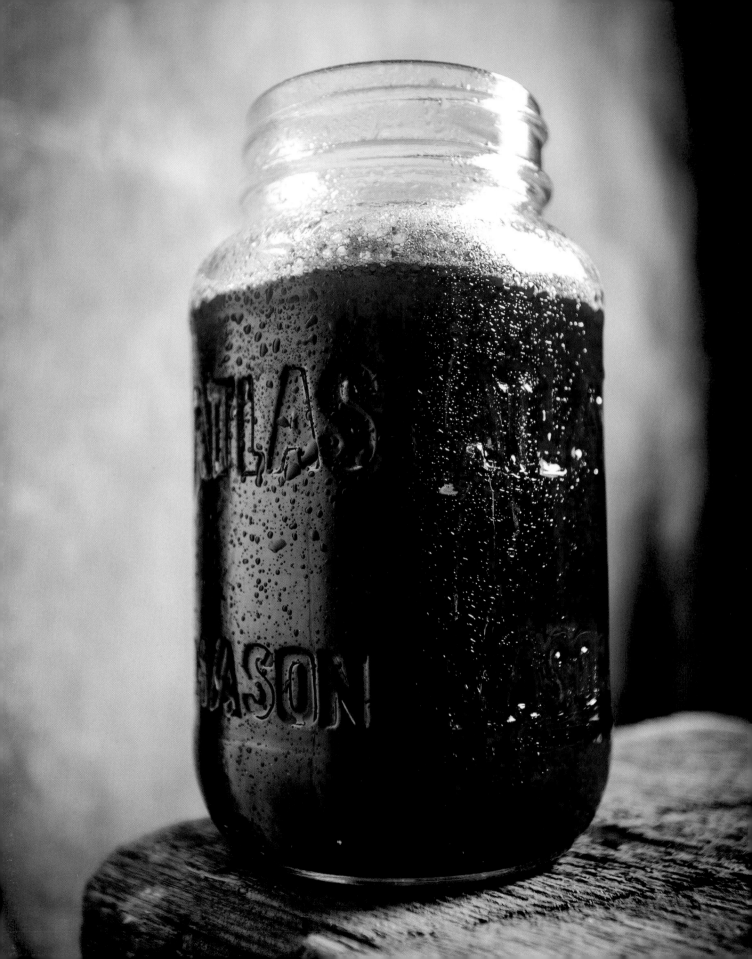

GINGER NITROUS

The beet is packed with nitrates that the body converts into nitrous oxide, thereby enhancing blood flow, so this juice will have you quickly absorbing its nutrition and feeling the rush of the ginger. It's a great sustainable-energy booster and a perfect replacement for coffee. Serves 1/Makes 1¾ cups (425 mL)

 Raw   Gluten-Free   **SND** Super Nutrient-Dense

Prep Time: 4 to 5 minutes • **Special Equipment:** high-speed juicer

Juice the beet, apple, carrot, and ginger in a high-speed juicer. Stir in the orange juice, lemon juice, and tea powder mix.

. . . .

• You can always add more ginger if you like. In my opinion, the more the better!

1 medium or large red beet, peeled

1 medium or large apple, peeled

1 medium carrot, peeled and cut in half lengthwise

½-inch (1 cm) knob of fresh ginger, peeled

¼ cup (60 mL) freshly squeezed orange juice

1 tbsp (15 mL) freshly squeezed lemon juice

½ tsp (2 mL) ginger citrus tea powder mix (page 216)

glorious green shot

nectarine-pineapple perfection
(made with white nectarines)

aloe-ginger-pomegranate shot

ginger nitrous

nectarine-pineapple perfection

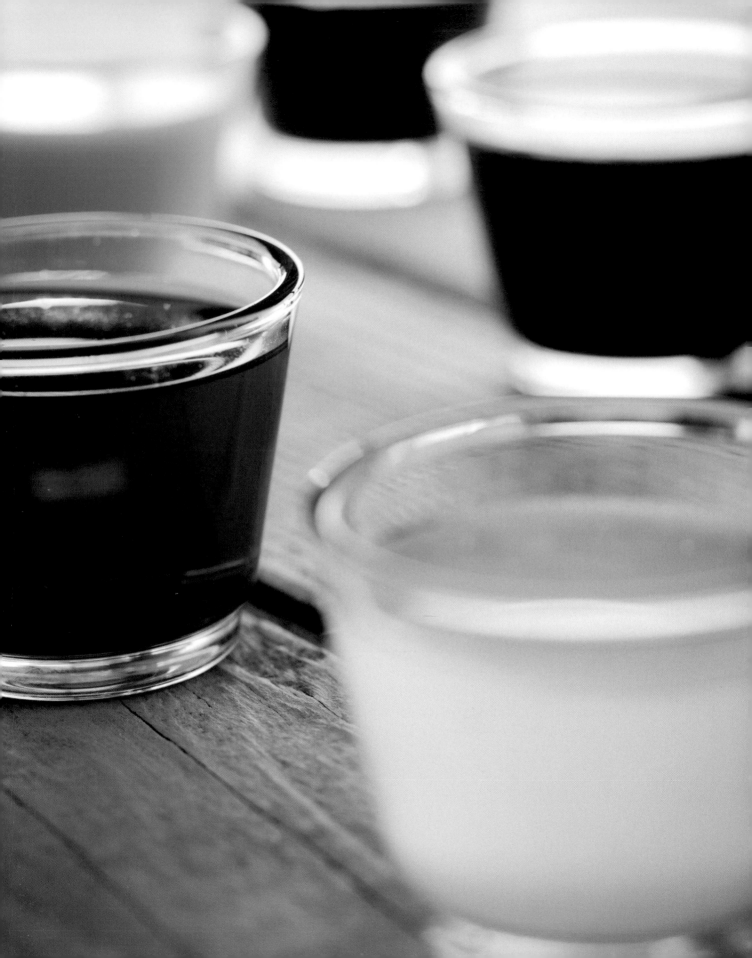

GREAT GREEN PICK-ME-UP

A simple combination of fresh and refreshing flavors, this is an ideal juice for the warm months—but delicious year round! Serves 1/Makes 1¾ cups (425 mL)

 Raw　　 Gluten-Free　　**SND** Super Nutrient-Dense

Prep Time: 3 to 4 minutes • **Special Equipment:** high-speed juicer

Juice all the ingredients in a high-speed juicer. This juice is best served chilled.

1 large green apple (unpeeled)

½ large or 1 medium English cucumber (unpeeled)

1 cup (250 mL) chopped fennel

2 tsp (10 mL) lime juice

NECTARINE-PINEAPPLE PERFECTION

With an invigorating combination of fresh flavors, this drink will aid in digestion because of the papain enzyme in the pineapple. Serves 1/Makes 1¾ cups (425 mL)

R Raw　　**GF** Gluten-Free

Prep Time: 3 to 4 minutes • **Special Equipment:** high-speed juicer

Juice the nectarines and pineapple in a high-speed juicer. Stir in the lime juice. This juice is amazing served cold!

2 nectarines, pitted and chopped

2 cups (500 mL) chopped pineapple

Juice of 1 lime

AMINO SUPER-SPROUT

Rich in amino acids, this refreshing juice of fresh shoots will give you a rush that feeds the cells and won't tax the adrenals. Serves 1/Makes 2¼ cups (550 mL)

 R Raw   **GF** Gluten-Free   **SND** Super Nutrient-Dense

Prep Time: 3 to 4 minutes
Special Equipment: slow-speed juice extractor, high-speed juicer

2 cups (500 mL) sunflower sprouts

2 cups (500 mL) pea shoots

Handful of fresh parsley

½ large English cucumber (unpeeled)

½ Bartlett pear

2 celery ribs

2 tbsp (30 mL) freshly squeezed lemon juice

Juice the sunflower sprouts, pea shoots, and parsley in a slow-speed juice extractor. Juice the cucumber, pear, and celery in a high-speed juicer.

Stir together the two juices and stir in the lemon juice.

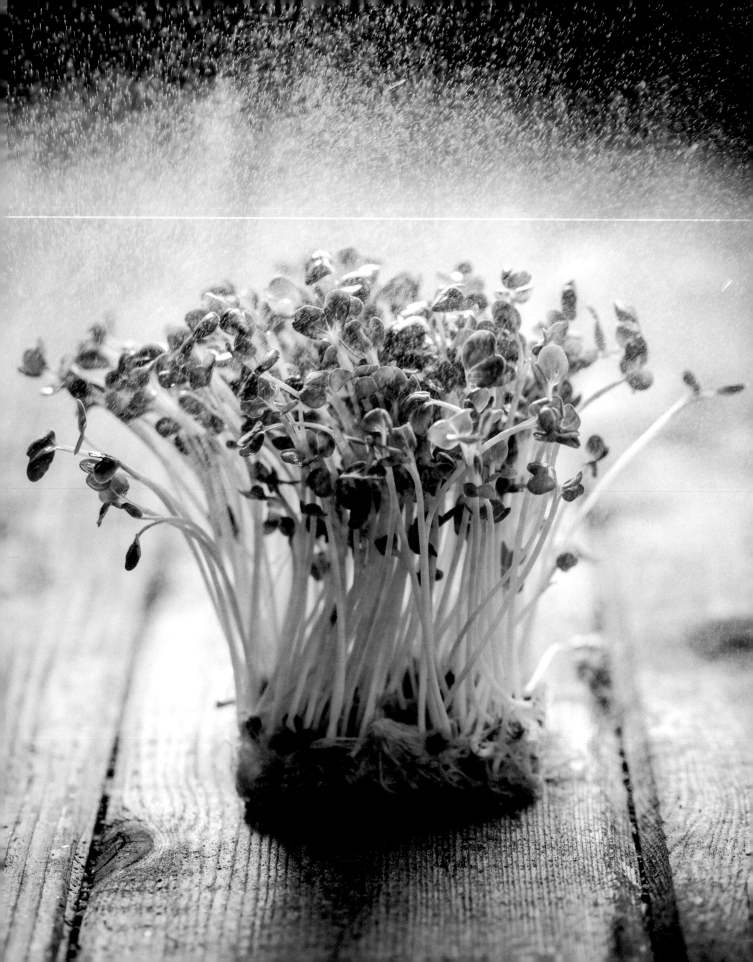

RADICAL RED TOMATO JUICE

A fresh, healthy twist on a classic. Minerals from the celery help replenish electrolytes and therefore help increase range of motion and facilitate smooth muscle contractions. Serves 1/Makes 1¾ to 2 cups (425 to 500 mL)

 Raw ● GF Gluten-Free ● SND Super Nutrient-Dense

Prep Time: 3 to 4 minutes • **Special Equipment:** high-speed juicer

Juice the tomato, celery, carrot, and cucumber in a high-speed juicer. Add the lime juice, Worcestershire sauce (if using), and salt and pepper to taste. Stir.

• A nice option is to lightly rim the glass with lime and pink Himalayan salt.

1 large ripe tomato

2 celery ribs

1 carrot, trimmed and peeled

⅓ English cucumber (unpeeled)

1 tbsp (15 mL) freshly squeezed lime juice

½ tsp (2 mL) organic Worcestershire sauce (optional)

Finely ground Himalayan pink salt and freshly ground black pepper

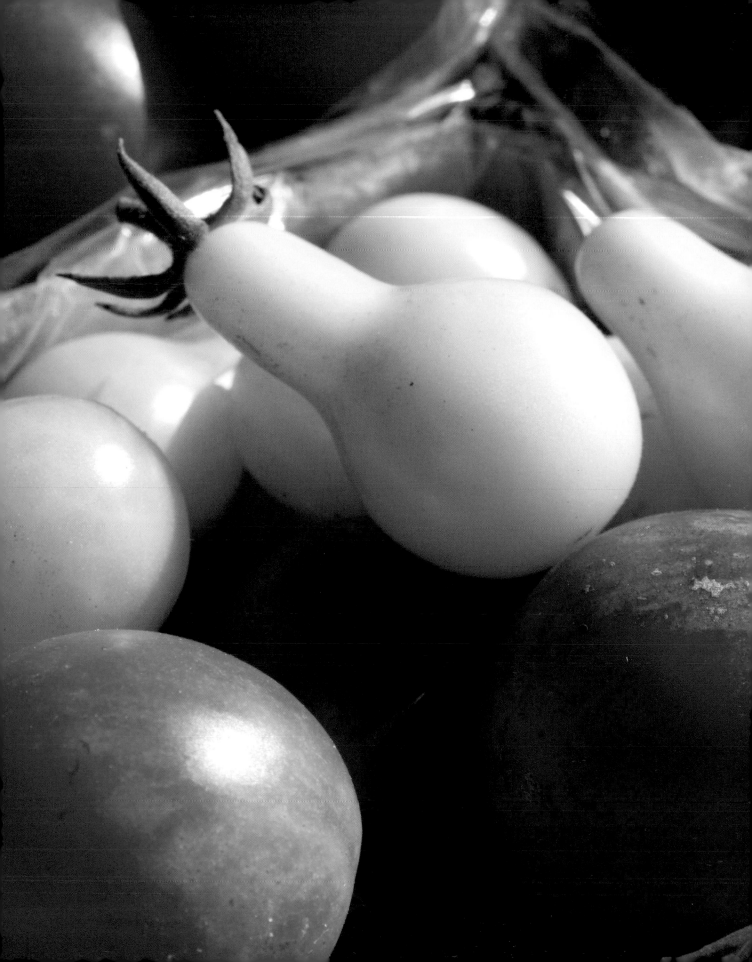

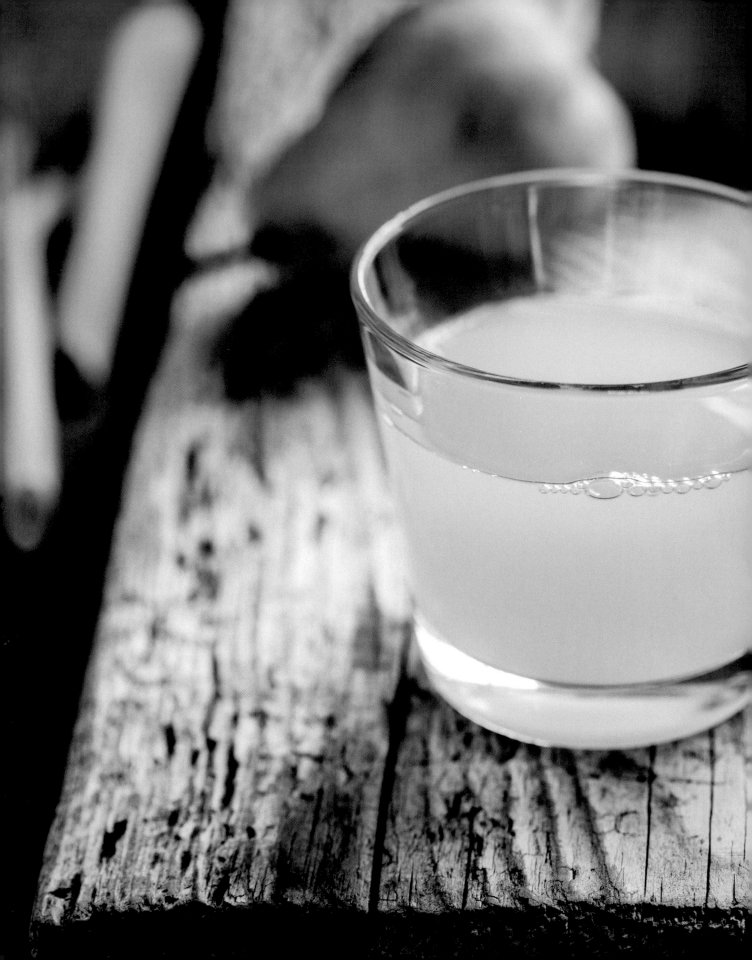

PEAR-GINGER-LEMONGRASS REFRESHER

Alkalinizing and refreshing, this drink will help reduce inflammation while hydrating. Serves 1/Makes 1¾ cups (425 mL)

T Transition   **GF** Gluten-Free

Prep Time: 3 to 4 minutes • **Special Equipment:** high-speed juicer

Cut off the bottom 6 inches (15 cm) or so of the lemongrass. Peel off and discard the tough outer leaves. Pound the lemongrass with the side of a large knife until its aromas are released. Set aside.

Juice the pears, apple, and ginger in a high-speed juicer. Pour into a glass and stir with the lemongrass stalk. Let lemongrass sit in the juice and refrigerate for 10 to 15 minutes to infuse and cool.

1 stalk lemongrass

2 pears

1 apple (unpeeled)

½-inch (1 cm) knob of fresh ginger

. . . .

• Use a pineapple wedge for garnish, if you like.

PINK WATERMELON GRAPEFRUIT COOLER

Simple and refreshing, this is the perfect summer drink. Serves 1/Makes 1¾ cups (425 mL)

R Raw   **GF** Gluten-Free

Prep Time: 3 to 4 minutes • **Special Equipment:** high-speed juicer

Bunch the mint up and juice it between the watermelon and grapefruit in a high-speed juicer.

Small handful of fresh mint leaves

2 cups (500 mL) cold chopped watermelon

1 pink grapefruit, peeled

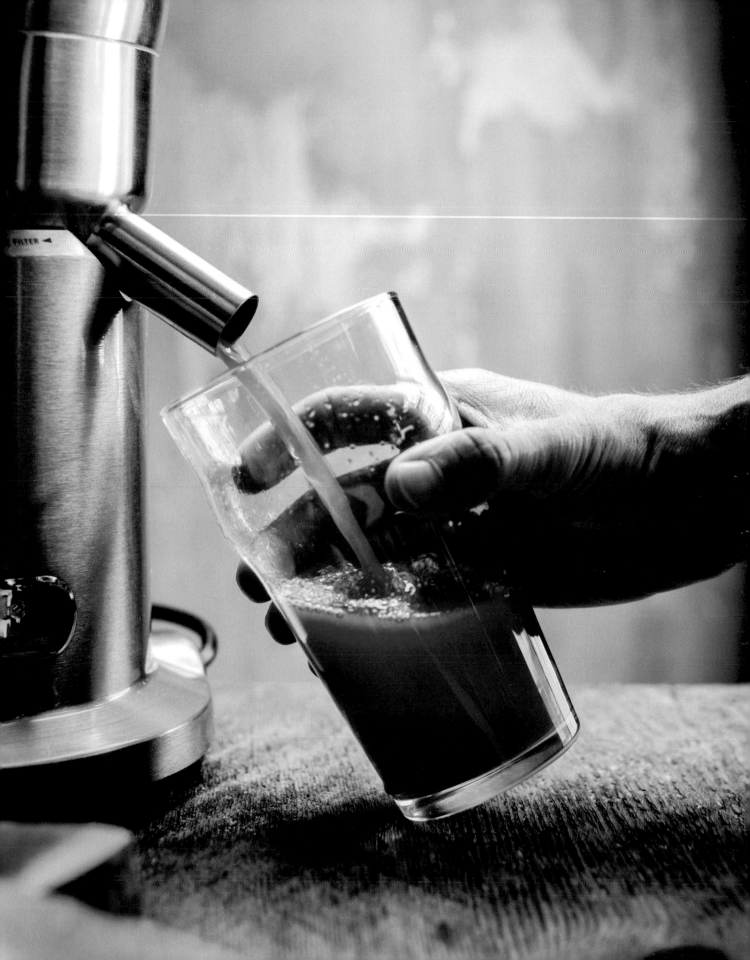

ALOE-GINGER-POMEGRANATE SHOT

This shot will enhance digestion and settle an upset stomach. You might pucker a little when you down it, but it's a great way to start off your day. Makes 2 single shots (4 oz/125 mL total)

 Raw   **GF** Gluten-Free   **SND** Super Nutrient-Dense

Prep Time: 4 to 5 minutes

2 tbsp (30 mL) aloe vera juice (from a whole leaf if possible)

1 tbsp (15 mL) freshly squeezed ginger juice

1 tbsp (15 mL) pure pomegranate juice

Stir together the three juices.

GLORIOUS GREEN SHOT

With its hefty dose of chlorophyll and minerals, this shot will help reduce inflammation. It's excellent right after a workout. Makes 2 single shots (4 oz/125 mL total)

R Raw   **GF** Gluten-Free   **SND** Super Nutrient-Dense

Prep Time: 4 to 5 minutes

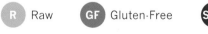

1 tbsp (15 mL) fresh wheat-grass juice

1 tbsp (15 mL) fresh parsley juice

1 tbsp (15 mL) fresh sunflower sprout juice

1 tbsp (15 mL) freshly squeezed lemon juice

Stir together all the ingredients. Drink immediately.

· ·

• **The best yield is obtained by slowly feeding in the wheatgrass.**

CHOCOLATE-TRUFFLE-CARAMEL MOCHA

A rich treat with a kick, this combination of ingredients delivers immediate and sustained energy—*and* it's delicious. Serves 1/Makes 1½ to 1¾ cups (375 to 425 mL)

T Transition   **GF** Gluten-Free

Prep Time: 3 to 4 minutes • **Special Equipment:** espresso maker

In a large mug, combine the lacuma powder, cacao powder, chocolate sauce, caramel sauce, vanilla, and agave. Stir into a paste. Add the espresso and top with the steamed almond milk. Garnish with more chocolate and caramel sauces, drizzling them on top of the almond foam in a zigzag pattern.

....

• For an optional garnish, sprinkle with cacao powder. It looks and tastes great.

1 tbsp (15 mL) lacuma powder

1 tsp (5 mL) cacao powder

1 tbsp (15 mL) chocolate sauce (page 215), plus more for garnish

1 tbsp (15 mL) lacuma caramel sauce (page 214), plus more for garnish

1 tsp (5 mL) pure vanilla extract

1 tsp (5 mL) agave nectar

1 or 2 shots espresso

1 cup (250 mL) unsweetened almond milk (or homemade, page 23), steamed

CINNAMON-SPICE ALMOND LATTE

This latte provides a blood-sugar-stabilizing kick, ideal for transitioning away from coffee. Serves 1/Makes 1½ to 1¾ cups (375 to 425 mL)

T Transition **GF** Gluten-Free

Prep Time: 3 to 4 minutes • **Special Equipment:** espresso maker

1 tbsp (15 mL) pure vanilla extract

1 tsp (5 mL) agave nectar

½ tsp (2 mL) latte spice mix (page 217)

1 or 2 shots espresso

1 cup (250 mL) unsweetened almond milk (or homemade, page 23), steamed

Cinnamon or nutmeg, for garnish

In a large mug, combine the vanilla, agave, and latte spice mix. Stir into a paste. Add the espresso and top with the steamed almond milk. Garnish with cinnamon or nutmeg—or try both!

MAYAN-SPICED HOT CHOCOLATE

A warming, adrenal-nourishing, and nutrient-rich update of a classic. The optional cayenne is recommended because it increases blood flow and therefore speeds the absorption of nutrients. Serves 1/Makes 1½ to 1¾ cups (375 to 425 mL)

 Gluten-Free   **SND** Super Nutrient-Dense

Prep Time: 3 to 4 minutes • **Special Equipment:** espresso maker

In a large mug, combine all the ingredients except the coconut milk and almond milk. Stir into a paste. Stir in the coconut milk. Top with the steamed almond milk. Garnish with more chocolate sauce, drizzling it on top of the almond foam in a zigzag pattern.

....

• For a different garnish, sprinkle with cacao powder.

1 tbsp (15 mL) spiced hot chocolate powder (such as Camino brand)

1 tbsp (15 mL) chocolate sauce (page 215), plus more for garnish

1 tsp (5 mL) cacao powder

½ tsp (2 mL) maca powder

⅛ tsp (0.5 mL) cayenne pepper (optional)

2 tbsp (30 mL) hot water

1 tsp (5 mL) pure vanilla extract

1 tsp (5 mL) agave nectar or maple syrup (or stevia for low carb)

½ tsp (2 mL) latte spice mix (page 217)

2 tbsp (30 mL) coconut milk

1 cup (250 mL) unsweetened almond milk (or homemade, page 23), steamed

VANILLA-ALMOND CHAI LATTE

Simple and warming, this drink is perfect for the colder months. Serves 1/Makes 1½ to 1¾ cups (375 to 425 mL)

 Gluten-Free

Prep Time: 3 to 4 minutes • **Special Equipment:** espresso maker

In a large mug, steep the tea bag in the hot water for 2 to 3 minutes. Stir in the vanilla, latte spice mix, and agave. Remove the tea bag. Top with the steamed almond milk and dust with some latte spice mix.

1 chai tea bag

¼ cup (60 mL) hot water

1 tsp (5 mL) pure vanilla extract or powder

½ tsp (2 mL) latte spice mix (page 217), plus more for garnish

½ tsp (2 mL) agave nectar or maple syrup (or stevia for low carb)

1 cup (250 mL) unsweetened almond milk (or homemade, page 23), steamed

ZEN MATCHA TEA MISTO

This phytochemical-rich coffee substitute is a Thrive Energy favorite of the on-the-way-to-yoga crowd. Serves 1/Makes 1¾ cups (425 mL)

 Gluten-Free   **SND** Super Nutrient-Dense

Prep Time: 3 to 4 minutes • **Special Equipment:** espresso maker

In a large mug, combine the matcha powder, vanilla, and agave. Stir into a paste. Add the hot water and stir to dissolve all the ingredients. Top with the steamed milk and dust with some matcha powder.

1 tbsp (15 mL) matcha power, plus more for garnish

1 tsp (5 mL) pure vanilla extract or powder

1 tsp (5 mL) agave nectar or maple syrup (or stevia for low carb)

¼ cup (60 mL) hot water

1 cup (250 mL) unsweetened almond milk (or homemade, page 23), steamed

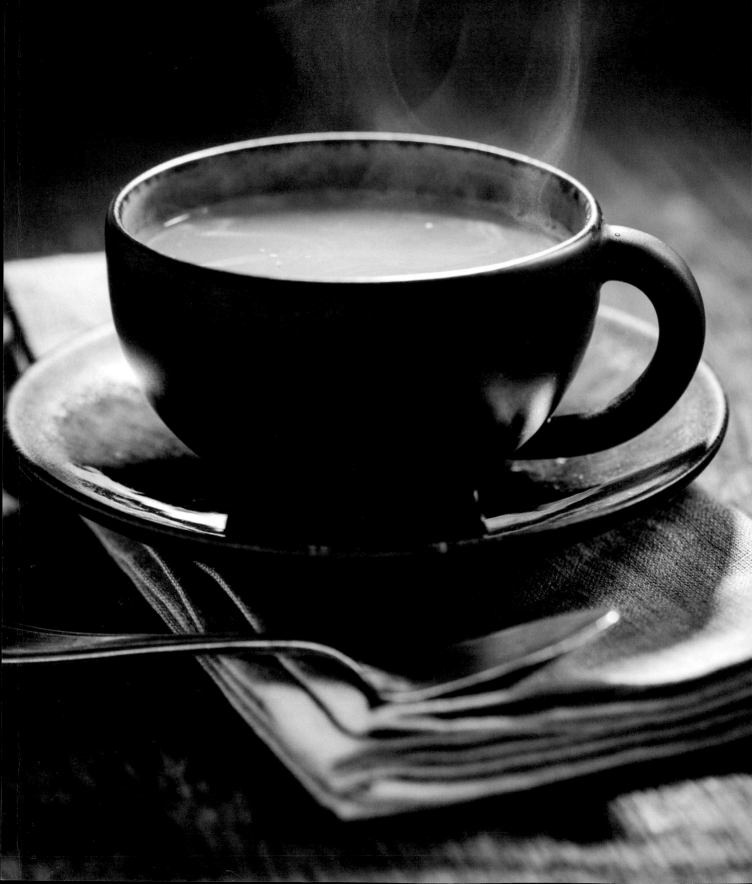

GINGER-CITRUS TEA INFUSION

A delicious and refreshing anti-inflammation coffee alternative. Serves 1/Makes 1½ to 1¾ cups (375 to 425 mL)

 GF Gluten-Free

Prep Time: 5 minutes
Special Equipment: espresso maker with steam wand, slow-speed juice extractor

Juice the ginger in a slow-speed juice extractor. In a large mug, combine the ginger juice, orange juice, lemon juice, tea powder mix, vanilla, and agave. Steam until slightly frothy but do not boil. Stir in the hot water.

1 tbsp (15 mL) chopped fresh ginger, or more to taste

6 tbsp (90 mL) freshly squeezed orange juice

3 tbsp (45 mL) freshly squeezed lemon juice

1 tsp (5 mL) ginger citrus tea powder mix (page 216)

1 tsp (5 mL) pure vanilla extract or powder

1 tsp (5 mL) agave nectar or maple syrup (or stevia for low carb)

1 cup (250 mL) hot water

LACUMA CARAMEL SAUCE

A smooth functional sauce, rich in vitamins and minerals, designed to help those transitioning to a cleaner diet while not neglecting their sweet tooth. Makes 2 cups (500 mL)

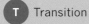 Transition   GF Gluten-Free

Prep Time: 4 to 5 minutes • **Special Equipment:** high-speed blender

¾ to 1 cup (175 to 250 mL) warm water

1 cup (250 mL) raw cashew butter

⅔ cup (150 mL) agave nectar or maple syrup

2 tbsp (30 mL) lacuma powder

1 tbsp (15 mL) pure vanilla extract or powder

Pinch of sea salt

Place 2 tbsp (30 mL) of the water in a blender. Add the remaining ingredients. Blend until thick but pourable, adding more water if needed.

• Best stored in a squeeze bottle.
• Keeps in a sealed container, refrigerated, for up to 3 weeks. The sauce thickens when it's cold, so take it out of the fridge at least a half-hour before using.

CHOCOLATE SAUCE

A healthy update to the classic chocolate sauce, this easy version is as rich as the traditional version yet provides several nutritional advantages. It's a great smoothie topping for those who are transitioning to a cleaner diet. Makes 2 cups (500 mL)

R Raw   **T** Transition   **GF** Gluten-Free

Prep Time: 5 minutes • Special Equipment: blender

Blend all the ingredients in a blender until smooth.

• Keeps in the fridge for 4 to 5 days.

1 cup (250 mL) cacao powder

½ cup (125 mL) coconut oil (melted)

½ tsp (2 mL) sea salt

½ cup (125 mL) agave nectar

3 tbsp (45 mL) water

BIG ORANGE SMOOTHIE POWDER MIX

Immune-boosting, inflammation-reducing, and adrenal-nourishing, this powder packs a nutritional punch and has a distinctive earthy flavor.

 Gluten-Free   Super Nutrient-Dense

Prep Time: 4 minutes • **Special Equipment:** spice grinder

1 part turmeric

1 part echinacea

1 part maca

1 part astragalus

Combine all the roots in a spice grinder and grind to a fine powder. If you're starting out with powdered ingredients, just stir them together.

....

• Keeps in a sealed container, in a cool, dry place, for several months.

GINGER CITRUS TEA POWDER MIX

Inflammation-reducing and immune-enhancing, this is a powerhouse of function. Stir it into warm drinks to boost their nutritional value.

 Gluten-Free   Super Nutrient-Dense

Prep Time: 4 minutes • **Special Equipment:** spice grinder

1 part astragalus

1 part ginseng

1 part echinacea

Combine all the roots in a spice grinder and grind to a fine powder. If you're starting out with powdered ingredients, just stir them together.

....

• Keeps at full potency, in a sealed container in a cool, dry place, for about 4 months.

LATTE SPICE MIX

This nutrient-dense flavor-blaster can be mixed into hot drinks to stabilize blood sugar.

 Gluten-Free

Prep Time: 4 minutes • **Special Equipment:** spice grinder

2 parts cinnamon

2 parts nutmeg

1 part cloves

Combine all the ingredients in a spice grinder and grind to a fine powder. If you're starting out with powdered ingredients, just stir them together.

....

• Keeps in a sealed container, in a cool, dry place, for at least 4 months.

SUPER CHOCOLATE POWDER MIX

This tasty powder is an absolute powerhouse of adrenal-restorative function. It dramatically enhances the nutritional value of any drink.

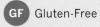 Gluten-Free SND Super Nutrient-Dense

---

Prep Time: 4 minutes • **Special Equipment:** spice grinder

Combine all the ingredients in a spice grinder and grind to a fine powder. If you're starting out with powdered ingredients, just stir them together.

1 part reishi mushroom

1 part cinnamon

1 part yerba mate

1 part ginseng

1 part maca

....

• Keeps in a sealed container, in a cool, dry place, for a long time, so make enough to last.

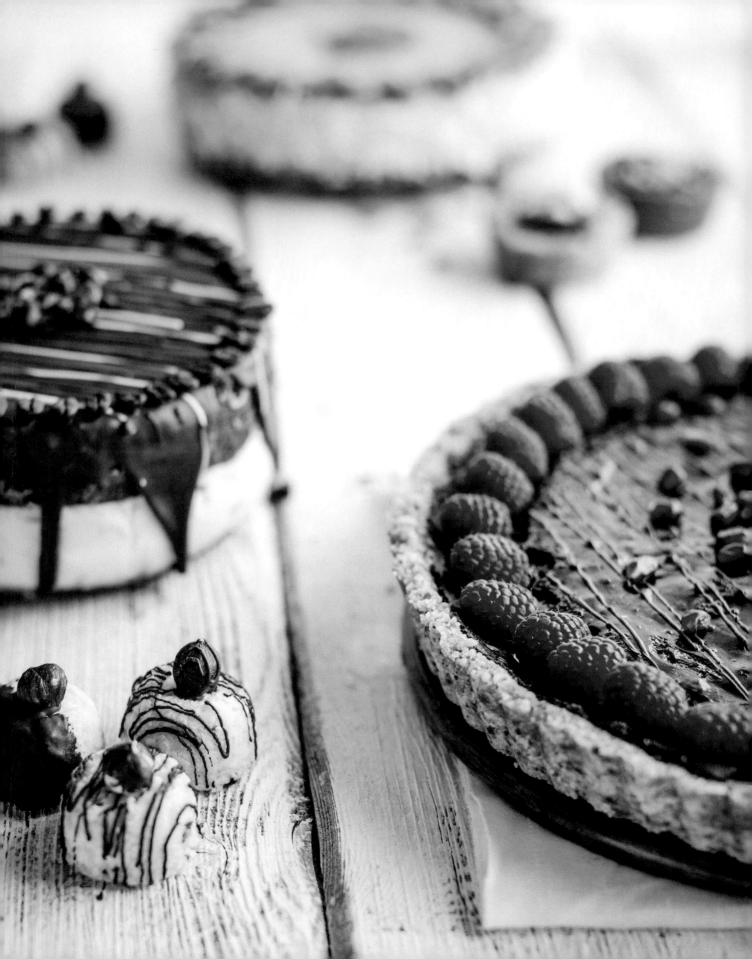

DESSERTS

BUCKWHEAT CHOCOLATE CHIP COOKIES

The cookies in this chapter, and the Pecan Bars on page 231, were designed to help with the transition from standard sweets and desserts to ones with nutritional value. From there, I suggest transitioning further to raw desserts such as the Nutty-Seed Cupcakes (page 235), Cashew Chocolate Mousse Layer Cake (page 244), and Raspberry Chocolate Pomegranate Tart (page 240). I've seen some people who have tried to make the jump from several decades of standard North American eating straight into clean, whole food eating, and it was simply too jarring for their body. So I believe these cookies serve as an excellent bridge to progressively better nutrition. Makes 14 cookies

 T Transition   **GF** Gluten-Free

Prep Time: 6 minutes • **Special Equipment:** stand mixer

4 tsp (20 mL) chia seeds

3 tbsp (45 mL) water

1 cup (250 mL) Earth Balance Vegan Buttery Sticks

1½ cups (375 mL) vegan cane sugar

2½ cups (625 mL) buckwheat flour

1 tsp (5 mL) baking soda

1 tsp (5 mL) sea salt

1 tsp (5 mL) cinnamon

1 cup (250 mL) vegan dark chocolate chips

½ cup (125 mL) walnuts, chopped

Preheat oven to 350°F (180°C). Line a baking sheet with parchment paper.

Stir together the chia seeds and water in a small bowl and allow to set up in the fridge. Meanwhile, in a stand mixer fitted with the paddle attachment, cream the butter with the sugar just until fluffy. Do not over-cream. Add the chia mixture; mix just until combined. Stir together the flour, baking soda, salt, and cinnamon. Add to the butter mixture and beat just until combined. Do not overmix. Stir in the chocolate chips and walnuts.

Using an ice-cream or cookie scoop, drop batter onto the baking sheet about 2 inches (5 cm) apart. Press down with your hand or a fork to flatten slightly.

Bake, rotating baking sheet halfway through, for 15 minutes or until cookies are firm to the touch. Let cool completely on the baking sheet.

....

• Over-creaming the butter and sugar will cause the cookies to spread too much.

BUCKWHEAT AMARANTH TRAIL MIX COOKIES

Another delicious recipe for those aiming to transition to cleaner eating habits. These cookies contain maca, which will help reduce cortisol levels, directly leading to reduced sugar cravings. Makes 14 cookies

T Transition   **GF** Gluten-Free

Prep Time: 8 minutes • **Special Equipment:** stand mixer

Preheat oven to 350°F (180°C). Line a baking sheet with parchment paper.

Stir together the chia seeds and water in a small bowl and allow to set up in the fridge.

Meanwhile, in a stand mixer fitted with the paddle attachment, cream the butter with the sugar just until fluffy. Do not over-cream. Add the chia mixture; mix just until combined.

Stir together the buckwheat flour, amaranth flour, baking soda, salt, and maca. Add to the butter mixture and beat just until combined. Do not overmix. Stir in the pumpkin seeds, sunflower seeds, coconut, cranberries, and pecans.

Using an ice-cream or cookie scoop, drop batter onto the baking sheet about 2 inches (5 cm) apart. Press down with your hand or a fork to flatten slightly.

Bake, rotating baking sheet halfway through, for 15 minutes or until cookies are firm to the touch. Let cool completely on the baking sheet.

4 tsp (20 mL) chia seeds

3 tbsp (45 mL) water

1 cup (250 mL) Earth Balance Vegan Buttery Sticks

1½ cups (375 mL) vegan cane sugar

2 cups (500 mL) light buckwheat flour

½ cup (125 mL) amaranth flour or quinoa flour

1 tsp (5 mL) baking soda

1 tsp (5 mL) sea salt

1 tsp (5 mL) maca root powder

¼ cup (60 mL) pumpkin seeds

¼ cup (60 mL) sunflower seeds

¼ cup (60 mL) unsweetened shredded coconut

¼ cup (60 mL) dried cranberries

¼ cup (60 mL) pecans, almonds, or walnuts, chopped

• **Over-creaming the butter and sugar will cause the cookies to spread too much.**

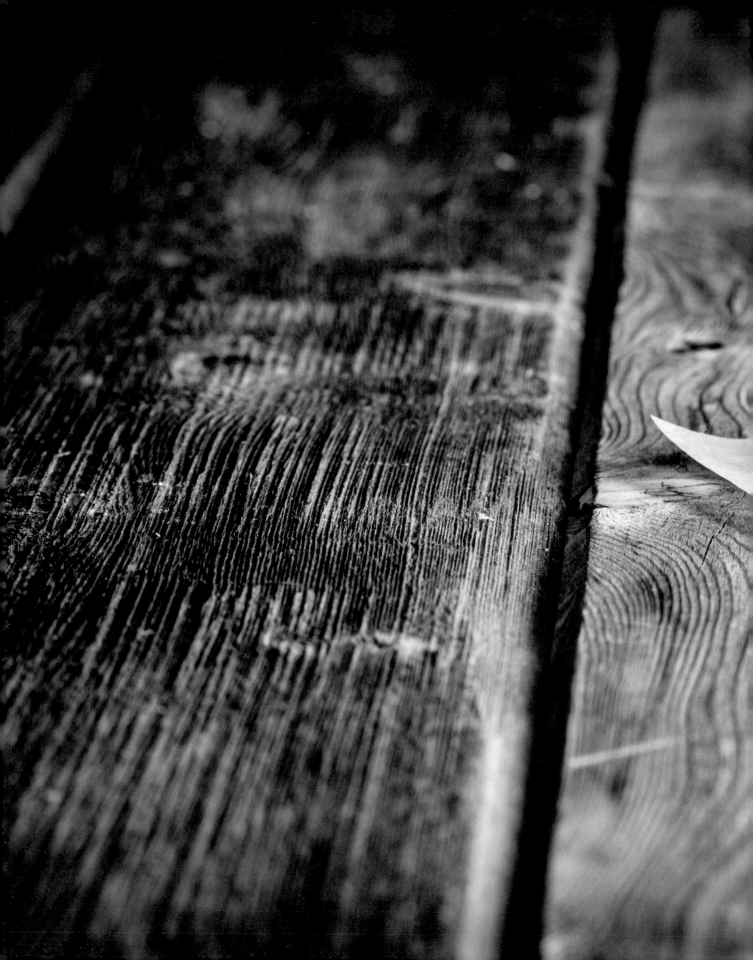

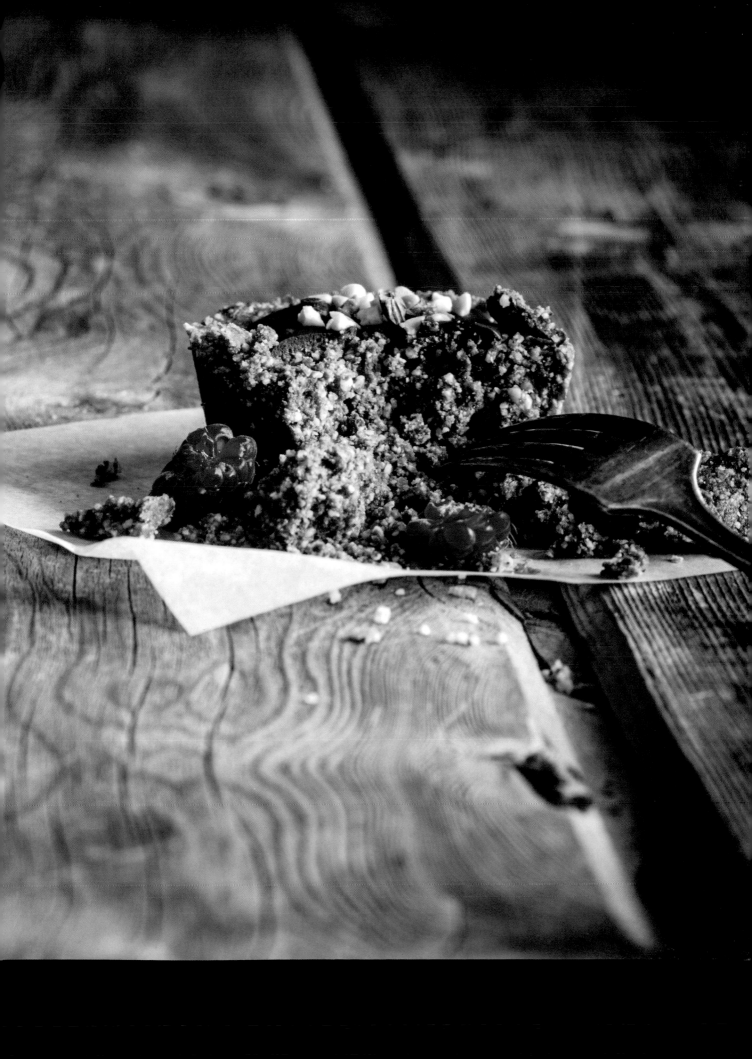

COCOA & ORANGE NUT COOKIES

These cookies not only taste great, they are functional flour-free cookies—nutritious and delicious cookies that really embrace a clean diet. Makes 11 to 14 cookies

 Gluten-Free   R Raw Option

Prep Time: 5 minutes, plus overnight soaking
Special Equipment: food processor, dehydrator (for raw version)

1½ cups (375 mL) pecans

1 cup (250 mL) almonds

½ cup (125 mL) cacao powder

¼ cup (60 mL) maple syrup or agave nectar

1 tbsp (15 mL) coconut oil

1 tsp (5 mL) pure vanilla extract

Pinch of sea salt

½ cup (125 mL) cacao nibs

1½ tbsp (22 mL) grated orange zest

1 cup (250 mL) chocolate ganache (page 40)

2 tbsp (30 mL) ground pistachios

Soak the pecans and almonds in water overnight.

Preheat oven to 250°F (120°C). Line a baking sheet with parchment paper.

Drain the nuts. In a food processor, process the nuts to a damp flour. Add the cacao powder, maple syrup, coconut oil, vanilla, and salt. Process until a dough forms. Transfer dough to a medium bowl and mix in the cacao nibs and orange zest by hand.

Form into 11 to 14 balls and place on the baking sheet about 2 inches (5 cm) apart. Press down with your hand to flatten slightly.

Bake, rotating baking sheet halfway through, for 1 hour or until cookies are firm to the touch. Let cool completely on the baking sheet.

Decorate with chocolate ganache and ground pistachios.

. . . .

- The cookies are baked at a low temperature to preserve the quality of the fats in the coconut oil.
- For a raw version of this cookie, instead of baking, dehydrate the cookies in a 115°F (46°C) dehydrator for 8 hours.

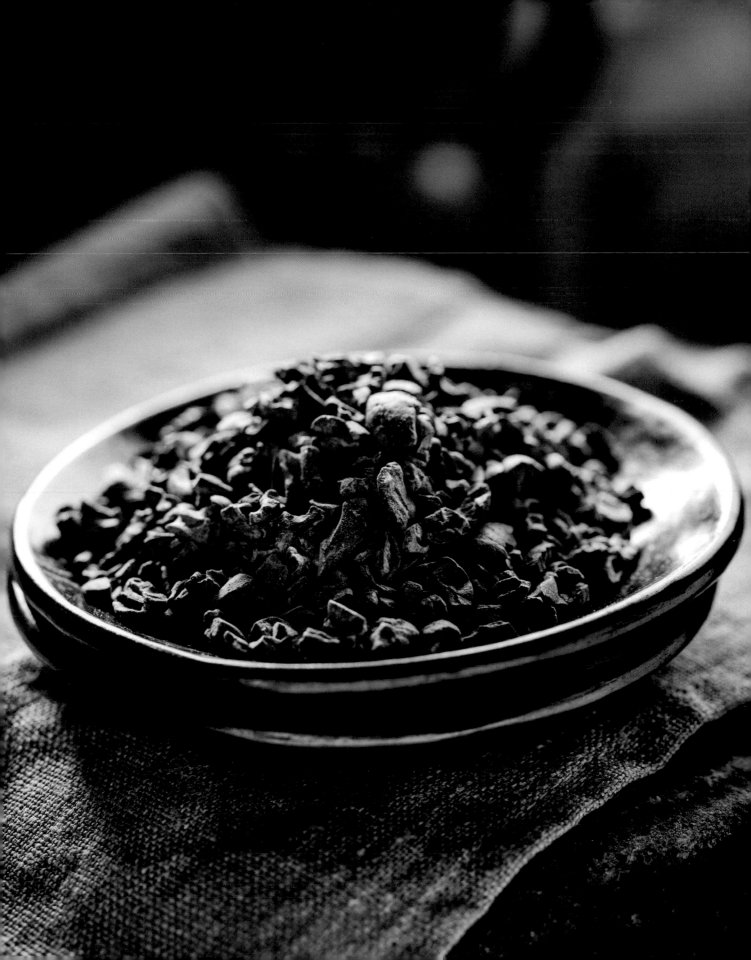

COCONUT PINEAPPLE MACAROONS

Made primarily from coconut, these macaroons are rich in high-quality fats that are easy to assimilate. Plus, digestion is aided by an enzyme called bromelain found in pineapple. Makes 18 to 20 macaroons

GF Gluten-Free   **R** Raw Option

Prep Time: 5 minutes • **Special Equipment:** food processor, dehydrator

4½ cups (1.125 L) unsweetened shredded coconut

¼ cup (60 mL) diced fresh pineapple

½ cup (125 mL) dried pineapple, finely chopped, plus more for garnish

½ cup (125 mL) maple syrup

2 tbsp (30 mL) coconut flour

1 tbsp (15 mL) vanilla powder or extract

¼ tsp (1 mL) sea salt

Chocolate ganache (page 40)

In a food processor, process 2½ cups (625 mL) of the shredded coconut until smooth and creamy, scraping down the sides regularly. This may take 5 to 10 minutes, depending on the power and speed of your food processor. Add the fresh pineapple and process until combined.

In a large bowl, combine the coconut purée, dried pineapple, coconut nectar, coconut flour, vanilla, and salt. Mix well. Add the remaining 2 cups (500 mL) shredded coconut and thoroughly combine with your hands.

Using a small or medium ice-cream or cookie scoop, measure equally sized portions of the macaroon mixture and arrange on a dehydrator tray or baking sheet.

Dehydrate at 108°F (42°C) for 24 hours (or bake on a parchment-lined baking sheet at 200°F/100°C for 20 to 30 minutes), until the macaroons are firm and dry to the touch. Let cool.

While the chocolate ganache is still viscous, use a spoon to drizzle it over the macaroons in a close zigzag pattern. (Alternatively, you can dip the macaroons into the chocolate.) Arrange the macaroons chocolate side up on the baking sheet. Garnish with a piece of dried pineapple, if desired, and refrigerate to set.

CHOCOLATE COCONUT MACAROONS

With a healthy kick of energy coming from good-quality fats in the coconut and chocolate, these macaroons are both functional and delicious. Makes 15 to 18 macaroons

 Gluten-Free

Prep Time: 5 minutes • **Special Equipment:** food processor, dehydrator

Macaroons

5 cups (1.25 L) unsweetened shredded coconut

½ cup (125 mL) maple syrup

2 tbsp (30 mL) coconut flour

2 tbsp (30 mL) cacao nibs

1 tbsp (15 mL) vanilla powder

¼ tsp (1 mL) sea salt

18 to 20 macadamia nuts, for garnish (optional)

Chocolate Ganache

½ cup (125 mL) thick fat from 1 can (14 oz/400 mL) coconut milk

4 tbsp (60 mL) Earth Balance Vegan Buttery Sticks

2 cups (500 mL) vegan dark chocolate chips

For the macaroons, in a food processor, process 3 cups (750 mL) of the shredded coconut until smooth and creamy, scraping down the sides regularly. This may take 5 to 10 minutes, depending on the power and speed of your food processor.

In a large bowl, combine the coconut purée, coconut nectar, coconut flour, cacao nibs, vanilla, and salt. Mix well. Add the remaining 2 cups (500 mL) shredded coconut and thoroughly combine with your hands.

Using a small or medium ice-cream or cookie scoop, measure equally sized portions of the macaroon mixture and arrange on a dehydrator tray or baking sheet. Dehydrate at 108°F (42°C) for 24 hours (or bake on a parchment-lined baking sheet at 200°F/100°C for 20 to 30 minutes), until the macaroons are firm and dry to the touch. Let cool.

For the ganache, in the top of a double boiler set over medium heat, heat the coconut milk and butter, stirring occasionally, until the butter is melted. Add the chocolate chips and stir until melted. Remove from heat and let cool slightly.

Line a baking sheet with waxed paper. While the chocolate is still viscous, use a spoon to drizzle it over the macaroons in a close zigzag pattern. (Alternatively, you can dip the macaroons into the chocolate.) Arrange the macaroons chocolate side up on the baking sheet. Garnish with a macadamia nut, if using, and refrigerate to set.

almond butter cups

blood orange
ginger citrus tart

coconut pineapple macaroons
and chocolate coconut macaroons

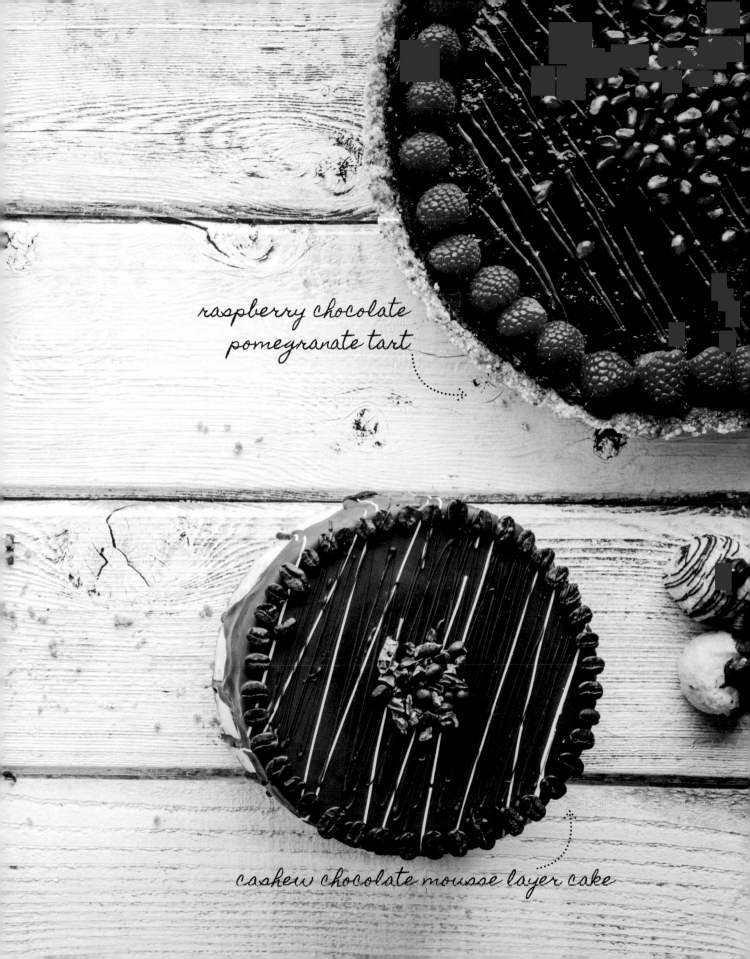

raspberry chocolate pomegranate tart

cashew chocolate mousse layer cake

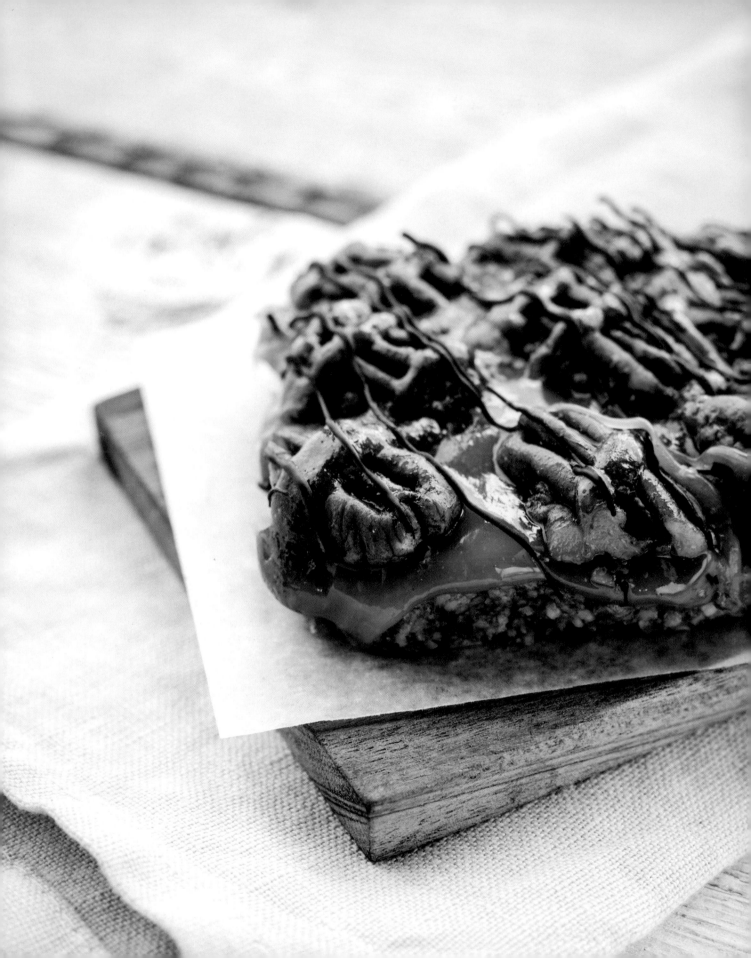

PECAN BARS

These bars were designed as a transitional dessert, moving away from conventional options laden with dairy and refined flour. While these are not as clean as the raw cakes in this chapter, they have developed a devout following among those aiming to phase out nutrient-devoid sweets and progress to healthier options.

Makes 15 squares

(T) Transition   (GF) Gluten-Free

Prep Time: 8 minutes, plus overnight chilling

Crust
2 cups (500 mL) brown rice flour

⅓ cup (75 mL) dark brown sugar

1 tsp (5 mL) sea salt

¼ tsp (1 mL) baking powder

¼ tsp (1 mL) cinnamon

¾ cup (175 mL) Earth Balance Vegan Buttery Sticks

Pecan Topping
2 cups (500 mL) coarsely chopped pecans

1½ cups (375 mL) dark brown sugar

⅔ cup (150 mL) coconut nectar

3 tbsp (45 mL) cornstarch

2 tbsp (30 mL) Earth Balance Vegan Buttery Sticks

2 tsp (10 mL) pure rum extract

¼ tsp (1 mL) sea salt

⅓ cup (75 mL) unsweetened almond milk (or homemade, page 23)

Preheat oven to 350°F (180°C). Line a 13- × 9-inch (3.5 L) cake pan with parchment paper, allowing a 2-inch (5 cm) overhang on two sides.

For the crust, in a large bowl, stir together the flour, brown sugar, salt, baking powder, and cinnamon. Use a pastry cutter or 2 knives to cut in the butter until the mixture resembles fine crumbs. Pour the crumbs into the prepared cake pan and press down evenly and very firmly, making sure to press the crumbs all the way to the edges of the pan.

Bake for 8 to 10 minutes, until firm and very lightly browned. Let cool on a rack.

For the topping, spread the pecans evenly over the crust. In a medium saucepan, heat the brown sugar, coconut nectar, cornstarch, butter, rum extract, and salt, stirring, until just bubbling. Remove from heat and stir in the almond milk. Pour over the pecans, making sure the topping is spread evenly.

Bake for 25 to 30 minutes or until bubbly. Let cool on a rack, then refrigerate overnight. Remove from the pan and cut into 15 bars.

. . . .

• These guys are really sticky and delicious so be sure to use parchment paper!

ALMOND BUTTER CUPS

These little treats are a delicious raw, nutrient-dense twist on the classic peanut butter cup. Makes 12 cups

T Transition   **GF** Gluten-Free

Prep Time: 10 minutes • **Special Equipment:** food processor

Crust

3 cups (750 mL) almonds

1 cup (250 mL) walnuts

¼ cup (60 mL) cacao nibs

6 Medjool dates, pitted, chopped, and soaked

3 tbsp (45 mL) agave nectar, maple syrup, or coconut nectar

Filling

⅓ cup (75 mL) virgin coconut oil, melted

⅓ cup (75 mL) almond butter (page 26)

⅓ cup (75 mL) agave nectar, maple syrup, or coconut nectar

¼ cup (60 mL) almond milk (page 23)

1 tsp (5 mL) pure vanilla extract

Topping

Chocolate sauce (page 215)

Garnish

¼ cup (60 mL) sliced almonds

¼ cup (60 mL) cacao nibs

For the crust, in a food processor, combine the almonds and walnuts. Process until the nuts are in very small pieces. Add the cacao nibs; pulse until they are the same size as the nuts. Add the dates and agave; pulse until a dough forms. Press the dough into the bottom and up the sides of 12 silicone cupcake molds, keeping it thin to ensure lots of room for the filling. Set aside.

For the filling, in a blender, combine all the ingredients. Process until smooth. Divide the filling among the molds. Refrigerate until firm, about 1 hour.

Spoon topping over the molds. Garnish with sliced almonds and cacao nibs.

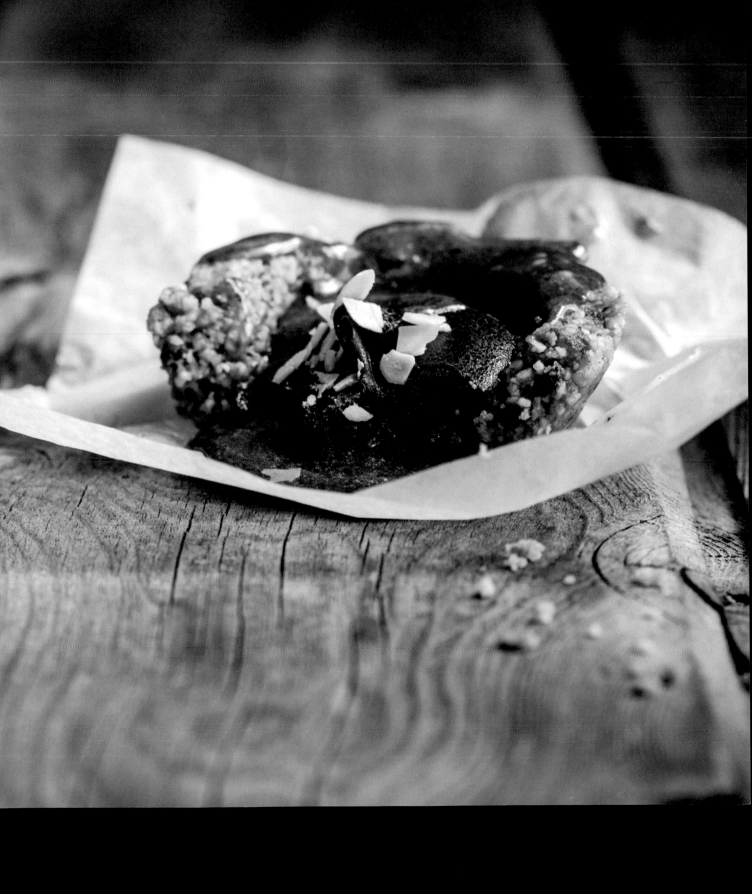

CHOCOLATE CACAO CUPCAKES

A decadent yet balanced blend of chocolate and cacao, combining sweet and slightly bitter, but all chocolate. These cupcakes are a good option for those transitioning to a cleaner plant-based diet. Makes 22 to 24 cupcakes

 Transition   GF Gluten-Free

Prep Time: 8 minutes

2 cups (500 mL) vegan cane sugar

2 cups (500 mL) almond milk (page 23)

2 tbsp (30 mL) cider vinegar

2 tsp (10 mL) pure vanilla extract

1 cup (250 mL) sorghum flour

½ cup (125 mL) quinoa flour

1 cup (250 mL) chickpea flour

¾ cup (175 mL) corn starch

¼ cup (60 mL) shredded unsweetened coconut

⅔ cup (150 mL) cacao powder

2 tsp (10 mL) baking soda

1½ tsp (2 mL) sea salt

⅔ cup (150 mL) virgin coconut oil, melted

Icing (pages 236 to 237)

Cacao nibs and shredded coconut, for garnish

Arrange racks in upper and lower thirds of oven and preheat oven to 350°F (180°C). Line two 12-cup muffin pans with paper liners.

In a large bowl, combine the cane sugar, almond milk, vinegar, and vanilla. In a medium bowl, sift together the flours, coconut, cacao powder, baking soda, and salt. Add the wet ingredients to the dry ingredients and stir until combined. Gently fold in the melted coconut oil until the batter is shiny and smooth but not overmixed. Spoon into muffin cups.

Bake, switching and rotating pans halfway through, for 25 minutes or until a toothpick inserted in the center comes out clean. Transfer to a rack and let cool completely.

Frost with desired icing and garnish with cacao nibs and shredded coconut.

• Overmixing the batter results in too much gluten formation, which will result in tough cupcakes.

NUTTY-SEED CUPCAKES

Unlike traditional versions made with refined flour, these cupcakes are functional and nutrient-dense. They are exceptionally filling, and so eating too many is difficult, just as it should be. Some people find half a cupcake is enough.

Makes 12 large cupcakes

R Raw   **GF** Gluten-Free

Prep Time: 6 minutes • **Special Equipment:** food processor

Combine all the ingredients except the icing in a food processor. Process until smooth.

Spoon the mixture into 12 muffin cups (or form the mixture into the shape of a cupcake and place on a baking sheet). Refrigerate for about 30 minutes to firm up. Frost with desired icing.

2 large Medjool dates, pitted

1 cup (250 mL) raw almonds

1 cup (250 mL) raw walnuts

½ cup (125 mL) raw sunflower seeds

¼ cup (60 mL) raw pumpkin seeds

¼ cup (60 mL) raw chia seeds

½ cup (125 mL) almond butter (page 26)

¼ cup (60 mL) coconut nectar or maple syrup

2 tsp (10 mL) pure vanilla extract

¼ tsp (1 mL) cinnamon

Icing (pages 236 to 237)

COCONUT LEMON ICING

A refreshing and satisfying twist on conventional icing, this one is made with a coconut-butter base and sweetened with clean-burning dates.

Makes about 1 cup (250 mL)

R Raw   **GF** Gluten-Free

Prep Time: 5 minutes • **Special Equipment:** blender

3 large Medjool dates, pitted and soaked

½ cup (125 mL) coconut butter (page 27)

¼ cup (60 mL) water

1 tbsp (15 mL) lemon zest

½ tsp (2 mL) pure vanilla extract

Combine all the ingredients in a blender. Blend until creamy, adding more water as needed for a smooth consistency.

• Keeps in a sealed container, refrigerated, for up to 2 weeks. Bring to room temperature before using.

CHOCOLATE AVOCADO ICING

You'll simply not believe this icing is made with only four ingredients, or that one of them is avocado. But it's nutritious and delicious, just the way functional icing should be. Makes 1½ cups (375 mL)

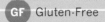 **GF** Gluten-Free

Prep Time: 5 minutes • **Special Equipment:** blender

Combine all the ingredients in a blender. Blend until creamy.

2 ripe avocados, peeled

¼ cup (60 mL) cacao powder

3 to 4 tbsp (45 to 60 mL) coconut nectar or maple syrup

Pinch of sea salt

• Keeps in a sealed container, refrigerated, for up to 2 weeks.

CHOCOLATE COCONUT ICING

Packed with clean-burning functional sugar from dates and high-quality usable fat from the coconut, this icing not only makes whatever you put it on taste better but also provides nutrition that's key to energy production. Ideal on long training days. Makes 1 cup (250 mL)

GF Gluten-Free

Prep Time: 5 minutes • **Special Equipment:** blender

Combine all the ingredients in a blender. Blend until creamy, adding a little more water if the icing is clumping. If necessary, refrigerate until icing is thick enough to spread.

6 large Medjool dates, pitted and soaked

¾ cup (175 mL) water

¼ cup (60 mL) raw cacao powder

¼ cup (60 mL) virgin coconut oil

• Keeps in a sealed container, refrigerated, for up to 2 weeks.

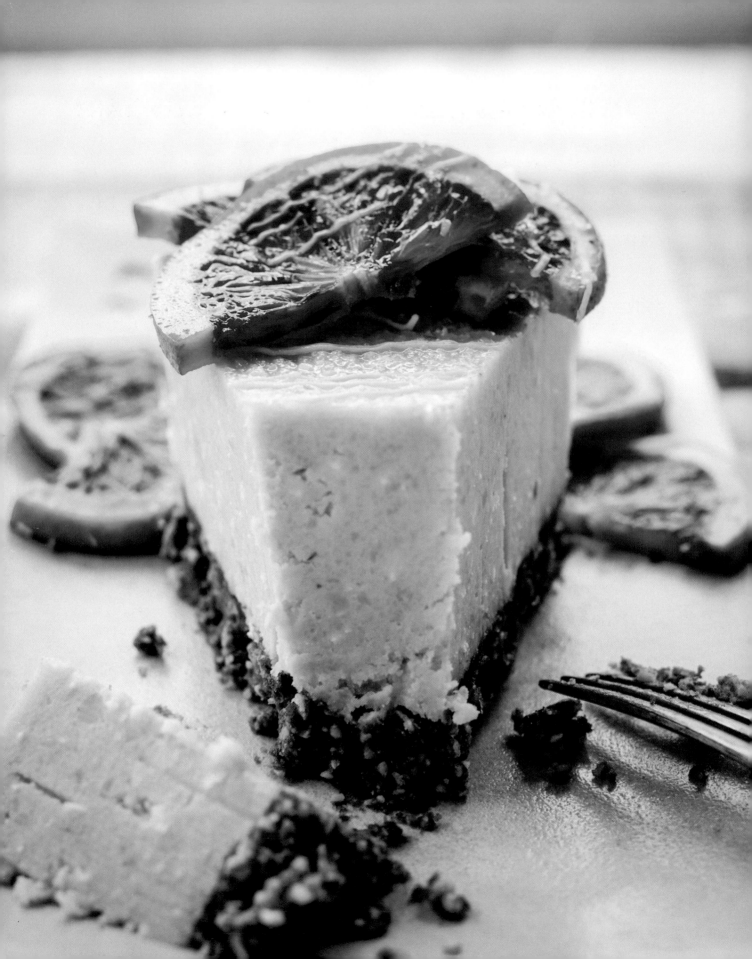

BLOOD ORANGE & GINGER CITRUS TART

A visually beautiful, decadent dessert that will satisfy your sweet tooth while helping to shift your palate toward simpler food combinations. Serves 6 to 8

T Transition   **GF** Gluten-Free

Prep Time: 20 minutes, plus overnight chilling
Special Equipment: nut mill or food processor

For the crust, in a medium bowl, combine the ground pecans, chopped almonds, almond meal, and cane sugar. Stir well. Rub in butter until well blended. Turn the crust mixture into a lightly greased 9-inch (2.5 L) springform pan and press firmly and evenly into the bottom. Cover and refrigerate for 1 hour.

Preheat oven to 350°F (180°C).

Bake the crust for 15 minutes. Let cool.

For the filing, in a medium saucepan, combine the sugar, cornstarch, and salt. Stir in the water and almond milk. Bring to a boil over medium heat, stirring, and cook, stirring constantly, until slightly thickened, 3 to 4 minutes. Remove from heat and stir in the orange zest, orange juice, and ginger juice. Pour into the cooled crust, cover, and refrigerate overnight.

Remove sides of pan and gently press the shredded coconut onto the sides of the tart. Arrange the orange slices around the top edge of the tart.

Drizzle the melted chocolate over the tart in a zigzag pattern from one side to the other.

- You can use any combination of nuts, such as hazelnuts or walnuts. Simply keep the overall nut ratio the same.
- If you can't find blood oranges, you can use any other type of orange.

Crust

2 cups (500 mL) finely ground pecans

1¾ cups (425 mL) finely chopped almonds

6 tbsp (90 mL) almond meal (flour)

3 tbsp (45 mL) brown cane sugar

¾ cup (175 mL) Earth Balance Vegan Buttery Sticks

Filling

1½ cups (375 mL) cane sugar

½ cup (125 mL) cornstarch

1 tsp (5 mL) salt

1¼ cups (300 mL) water

1 cup (250 mL) almond milk (page 23)

2 tbsp (30 mL) orange zest

¾ cup (175 mL) orange juice (from about 6 medium oranges)

1 tbsp (15 mL) ginger juice

Garnish

¼ cup (60 mL) unsweetened shredded coconut

2 blood oranges, sliced, each slice cut in half

¼ cup (60 mL) vegan white chocolate chips, melted

RASPBERRY CHOCOLATE POMEGRANATE TART

The classic flavor combination of raspberries and chocolate, combined with the antioxidant-rich pomegranate, make this dessert a functionally delicious powerhouse. Serves 6 to 8

 T Transition   **GF** Gluten-Free

Prep Time: 15 minutes, plus overnight chilling • **Special Equipment:** food processor

Crust

1 cup (250 mL) almonds

1 cup (250 mL) walnuts

3 tbsp (45 mL) cacao nibs

3 tbsp (45 mL) vegan dark chocolate chips

2 Medjool dates, pitted, chopped, and soaked

1 tsp (5 mL) pure vanilla extract

½ tsp (2 mL) sea salt

3 tbsp (45 mL) maple syrup

2 tbsp (30 mL) cacao butter or coconut oil, melted

Chocolate Ganache

2 small to medium avocados, peeled and pitted (do not use avocados that are too ripe)

½ cup (125 mL) cacao powder

2 tbsp (30 mL) almond or cashew butter

½ to ¾ cup (125 to 175 mL) maple syrup (optional)

¾ cup (175 mL) vegan semi-sweet chocolate chips, melted

1 tbsp (15 mL) pure vanilla extract

1 tsp (5 mL) sea salt

3 tbsp (45 mL) cacao butter or coconut oil, melted

Raspberry Pomegranate Filling

1½ cups (375 mL) fresh or frozen organic raspberries

¼ cup (60 mL) cane sugar or agave nectar

2 tbsp (30 mL) fresh lemon juice

2 tbsp (30 mL) pomegranate powder

2 tbsp (30 mL) pure pomegranate juice

1½ tbsp (22 mL) cornstarch

Garnish

½ cup (125 mL) pomegranate seeds

¼ cup (60 mL) vegan white chocolate chips, melted

¼ cup (60 mL) vegan dark chocolate chips, melted

½ cup (125 mL) fresh raspberries

¼ cup (60 mL) cacao nibs

For the crust, in a food processor, process the almonds, walnuts, cacao nibs, and chocolate chips until finely ground. Add the dates, vanilla, salt, maple syrup, and cacao butter; process until a sticky-to-touch dough forms. Press dough firmly into the bottom of a lightly greased 9-inch (2.5 L) springform pan. You should end up with a ½-inch (1 cm) thick crust. Save leftovers for up to one week in the fridge.

For the ganache layer, in the cleaned food processor, combine the avocados, cacao powder, almond butter, ½ cup maple syrup (if using), chocolate chips, vanilla, and salt. Process until smooth. Add the melted cacao butter while food processor is running. Blend until creamy and velvety. Taste and add the remainder of the maple syrup if you prefer the ganache sweeter. Scoop out this mixture and spread over the crust. Smooth out the top and refrigerate for about 30 minutes or until firm.

For the filling, in a medium saucepan bring all of the ingredients to a boil on medium to high heat. Keep stirring until the raspberries are dissolved. Strain the mixture over a bowl and discard the raspberry seeds. Set aside to cool.

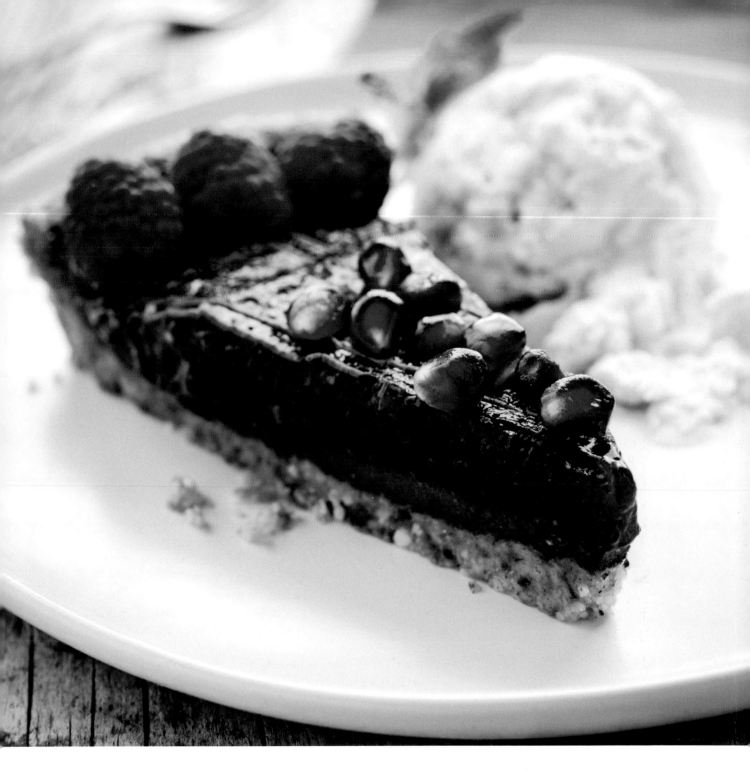

When the filling has cooled down, pour it over the chocolate ganache layer and smooth out the top. Cover and place in the freezer for 30 minutes to set.

To garnish, remove sides of pan. Drizzle the two kinds of melted chocolate over the tart in a zigzag pattern from one side to the other and allow the chocolate to drip down the sides. Spoon the pomegranate seeds and the cacao nibs onto the middle of the tart. Arrange the raspberries upside down around the edge of the tart.

STRAWBERRY, GOJI BERRY & DARK CHOCOLATE CHEESECAKE

This classically delicious textured cake—made completely flourless—has become hugely popular at the Thrive Energy Lab. Not only is it loved by traditional cake connoisseurs, it is rich in antioxidants, which come from the goji berries, and also has an above average amount of fiber for a cake because of the psyllium. Serves 8 to 10

(T) Transition   (GF) Gluten-Free

Prep Time: 20 minutes • **Special Equipment:** food processor, blender

Crust
1 cup (250 mL) raw almonds, soaked for 2 hours, rinsed

½ cup (125 mL) unsweetened coconut

¼ cup (60 mL) unsweetened cacao nibs

¼ cup (60 mL) cacao powder

⅓ cup (75 mL) Medjool dates, pitted

1 tsp (5 mL) vanilla extract

Pinch of sea salt

Cheesecake Base Layer
3 cups (750 mL) cashews, soaked for 2 to 4 hours, rinsed

1 cup (250 mL) dehydrated or dried strawberry pieces

½ cup (125 mL) dried goji berries, soaked for 1 hour, rinsed

⅓ cup (75 mL) lemon juice

¾ cup (175 mL) agave nectar

½ cup (125 mL) coconut oil, melted

1 tsp (5 mL) vanilla extract

½ tsp (2 mL) sea salt

2 cups (500 mL) fresh strawberries, diced

Chocolate Sauce
2 cups (500 mL) chocolate sauce (page 215)

Strawberry Coulis
2 cups (500 mL) fresh strawberries

¼ cup (60 mL) agave nectar

¾ tsp (4 mL) agar agar powder

1 tsp (5 mL) lemon juice

Pinch of sea salt

Garnish
1 cup (250 mL) fresh sliced strawberries

¼ cup (60 mL) dried goji berries

2 cups cacao nibs

For the crust, in a food processor, process the almonds, coconut, cacao nibs, and cacao powder until finely ground. Add the dates, vanilla, and salt; process until a sticky-to-touch dough forms. Press dough firmly into the bottom of a lightly greased 9-inch (2.5 L) springform pan. You should end up with a ½-inch (1 cm) thick crust. Save leftovers for up to one week in the fridge.

For the cheesecake base layer, process all of the ingredients except for the fresh strawberries in a food processor until smooth and creamy in texture. Then blend the fresh strawberries in a blender until smooth. Pour the fresh strawberry mixture into a fine mesh strainer and with a spatula press the mixture to get rid of some of the watery liquid. Save this for a smoothie later. Add the fresh pressed strawberry mixture to the cheesecake base layer mixture and mix together until well incorporated. Pour the mixture into a springform pan over the nut crust and smooth out the top with a knife or spatula. Refrigerate for 2 to 3 hours or more to set or place in the freezer overnight wrapped in cellophane.

Spread the chocolate sauce over the entire cheesecake with a long knife or a spatula, smoothing out at the end after you have covered the top and sides. If you prefer a thick chocolate topping, double the recipe and spread on a thicker layer.

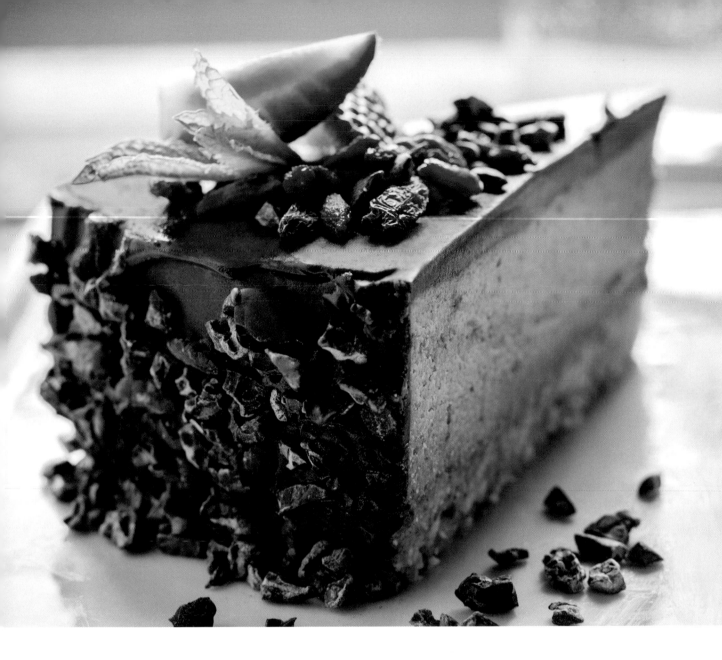

For the strawberry coulis, blend all of the ingredients together in a blender until smooth. Place mixture into a bowl and let chill in the fridge. Sauce will keep for at least one week in the fridge.

Gently rub a handful of cacao nibs over the sides of the cake, allowing the nibs to stick to the chocolate sauce. Don't worry about the pieces that fall off for now. After you've covered enough of the sides of the cake, you can use the remaining cacao nibs as decoration.

For the garnish, line the circumference of the cake with the sliced strawberries and sprinkle the center of the cake with the dried goji berries. Drizzle the strawberry coulis over each slice of cake and let it run down the sides. Serve chilled.

Stored in an airtight container, this cake will last up to 5 days.

CASHEW CHOCOLATE MOUSSE LAYER CAKE

A favorite for obvious reasons: this cake is delicious. Plus, it provides lasting nutrition from a variety of nuts. Ideally eaten on a day of high activity, it will help restock muscle glycogen levels by way of the agave nectar. Serves 8 to 12

(T) Transition   **(GF)** Gluten-Free

Prep Time: 10 minutes • Special Equipment: food processor

Crust

1 cup (250 mL) cashews

1 cup (250 mL) pecans

3 tbsp (45 mL) cacao nibs

¼ cup (60 mL) cacao powder

3 tbsp (45 mL) vegan dark chocolate chips

2 Medjool dates, pitted, chopped, and soaked

1 tsp (5 mL) pure vanilla extract

½ tsp (2 mL) sea salt

3 tbsp (45 mL) maple syrup

2 tbsp (30 mL) cacao butter or coconut oil, melted

Cashew Cake Layer

1 cup (250 mL) raw cashews, soaked for at least 6 hours, ideally overnight

½ cup (125 mL) hazelnuts, soaked for at least 6 hours, ideally overnight

1 tbsp (15 mL) fresh squeezed lemon juice

1 tsp (5 mL) pure vanilla extract

½ cup (125 mL) cacao butter or coconut oil, melted

½ cup (125 mL) agave nectar or maple syrup

Mousse Layer

3 small to medium avocados, peeled and pitted (do not use avocados that are too ripe)

½ cup (125 mL) cacao powder

2 tbsp (30 mL) almond or cashew butter

½ to ¾ cup (125 to 175 mL) maple syrup (optional)

1 tbsp (15 mL) pure vanilla extract

1 tsp (5 mL) sea salt

3 tbsp (45 mL) cacao butter or coconut oil, melted

¾ cup (175 mL) vegan semi-sweet chocolate chips, melted

Garnish

½ cup (125 mL) chocolate sauce (page 215)

1 cup (250 mL) whole raw cashews

Mint sprig

For the crust, in a food processor, process the cashews and pecans, cacao nibs, cacao powder, and chocolate chips until finely ground. Add the dates, vanilla, salt, maple syrup, and cacao butter; process until a sticky-to-touch dough forms. Press dough firmly into the bottom of a lightly greased 9-inch (2.5 L) springform pan. You should end up with a ½-inch (1 cm) thick crust. Save leftovers for up to one week in the fridge.

For the cake, blend the cashews and hazelnuts at medium speed for a few pulses. Add the remaining ingredients. Pulse at first and then run at high speed until desired texture and consistency are reached, which should take 3 to 5 minutes depending on the speed and power of your food processor. Remember to scrape down the walls when buildup occurs. Add water if needed until your filling tastes smooth and creamy.

With a spatula, scoop the mixture over the crust and smooth out the top. Cover with plastic wrap and place in the freezer for 30 minutes or until firm.

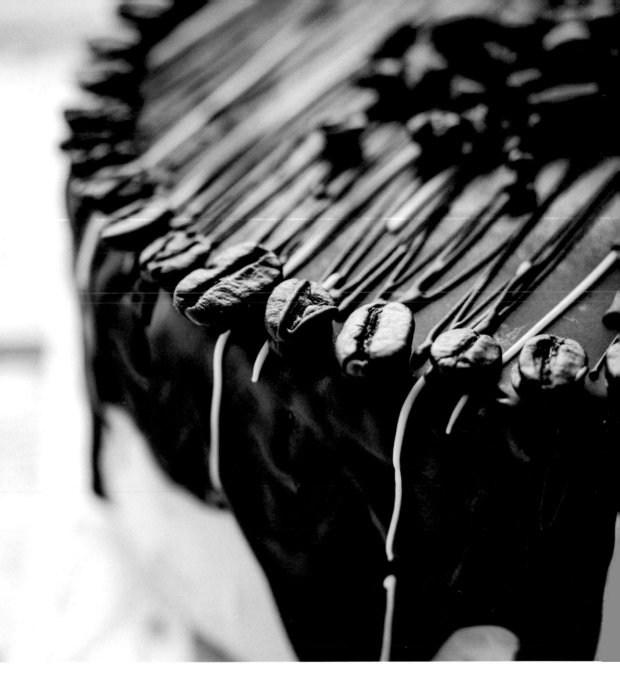

For the mousse layer, in the cleaned food processor, combine the avocados, cacao powder, almond butter, ½ cup maple syrup (if using), vanilla, and salt. Process until smooth. Add the melted cacao butter and the chocolate chips while food processor is running. Blend until creamy and velvety. Taste and add the remainder of the maple syrup if you prefer the mousse sweeter. Scoop out this mixture and spread the second layer over the cake. Smooth out the top and refrigerate for about 1 hour or until firm.

Carefully remove the sides of the pan and drizzle the chocolate sauce over the cake in a zigzag pattern from one side to the other, letting the sauce drip over the sides of the cake. Decorate the cake with the raw cashews around the circumference and a sprig of mint in the center.

CHOCOLATE-CHIA ICE CREAM WITH BLUEBERRIES

This has to be one of the simplest yet most delicious ice cream recipes there is. It contains no refined sugar, and the functional benefits of chia and maca make it an ideal dessert—or even a clean-burning addition to breakfast. Serves 4

 Transition   GF Gluten-Free   SND Super Nutrient-Dense   R Raw

---

Prep Time: 5 minutes • **Special Equipment:** food processor

Ice Cream

3 frozen bananas, sliced

2 large Medjool dates, pitted and soaked

1 tsp (5 mL) cocoa powder

2 tsp (10 mL) chia seeds

Blueberry Cream

1 banana

1 cup (250 mL) frozen blueberries

1 tsp (5 mL) maca (optional)

For the ice cream, in a food processor, combine all the ingredients. Process until creamy. Transfer to a bowl and place in the freezer.

Repeat with the blueberry cream ingredients. Add the blueberry cream to the ice cream and fold together just enough to leave swirls of blueberry. Serve immediately or freeze in an airtight container.

....

• Keeps, frozen, for several months. Let sit at room temperature for 10 minutes before serving.

CHOCOLATE CHIP, CHIA & MINT ICE CREAM

Everyone loves a chocolate-mint combination. With a tasty functional twist that includes chia seeds, this ice cream is a Thrive Energy winner. The optional green juice makes this alkaline-forming. Don't worry, you will not taste the greens.
Serves 4

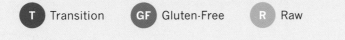

T Transition   **GF** Gluten-Free   **R** Raw

Prep Time: 5 minutes • **Special Equipment:** food processor

In a food processor, combine all the ingredients except the cacao nibs. Process until smooth. Stir in the cacao nibs. Serve immediately or freeze in an airtight container. Garnish with mint leaves, if desired.

• Keeps, frozen, for several months. Let sit at room temperature for 10 minutes before serving.

4 frozen bananas, sliced

¼ cup (60 mL) fresh mint leaves (about 10), plus more for garnish, if desired

1 tbsp (15 mL) green juice (optional)

1 tbsp (15 mL) coconut nectar (optional)

2 tsp (10 mL) chia seeds

½ tsp (2 mL) pure peppermint extract

½ tsp (2 mL) pure vanilla extract

Seeds scraped from 1 vanilla bean

Pinch of sea salt

2 tbsp (30 mL) raw cacao nibs

ORANGE, DATE & NUT CREAMSICLE

A nutrient-loaded twist on a classic flavor combination, this dessert has become a go-to favorite. Serves 4

GF Gluten-Free **R** Raw

Prep Time: 8 minutes • **Special Equipment:** food processor

4 frozen bananas, sliced

1 large Medjool date, pitted and soaked

2 tbsp (30 mL) finely chopped cashews

1 tbsp (15 mL) orange zest

1 tbsp (15 mL) fresh orange juice

1 tbsp (15 mL) coconut nectar (optional)

½ tsp (2 mL) pure vanilla extract

Seeds scraped from 1 vanilla bean

Pinch of sea salt

2 tbsp (30 mL) chopped cashews

In a food processor, combine all the ingredients except the chopped cashews. Process until smooth. Stir in the chopped cashews. Serve immediately or freeze in an airtight container.

....

• Keeps, frozen, for several months. Let sit at room temperature for 10 minutes before serving.

BERRY BLASTER ICE CREAM

With its creamy texture coming from the cashews, combined with the sweetness of the berries, it's hard to believe this ice cream is not only not bad for you but actually has many nutritional attributes, such as antioxidants, clean-burning carbohydrates, and raw healthy fats. Serves 4

 GF Gluten-Free   **R** Raw

Prep Time: 8 minutes • **Special Equipment:** food processor

In a food processor, combine all the ingredients except the raspberries. Process until smooth. Stir in the raspberries. Serve immediately or freeze in an airtight container.

....

• Keeps, frozen, for several months. Let sit at room temperature for 10 minutes before serving.

4 frozen bananas, sliced

1 large Medjool date, pitted and soaked

¼ cup (60 mL) frozen blueberries

2 tbsp (30 mL) finely chopped cashews

1 tbsp (15 mL) coconut nectar (optional)

½ tsp (2 mL) pure vanilla extract

Seeds scraped from 1 vanilla bean

Pinch of sea salt

¼ cup (60 mL) frozen raspberries, quartered

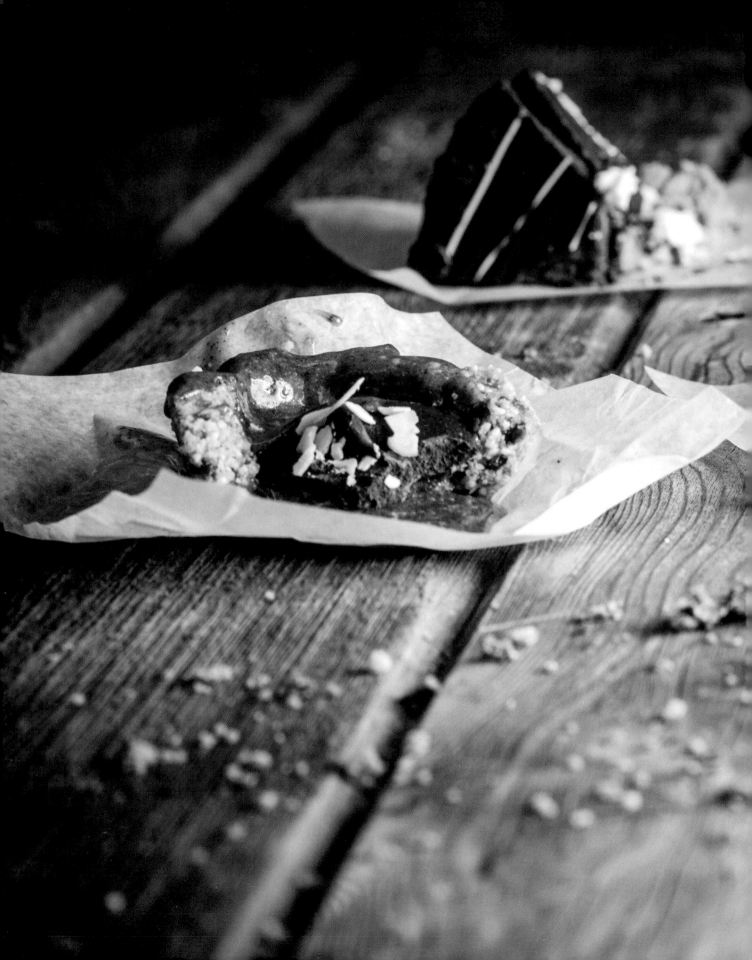

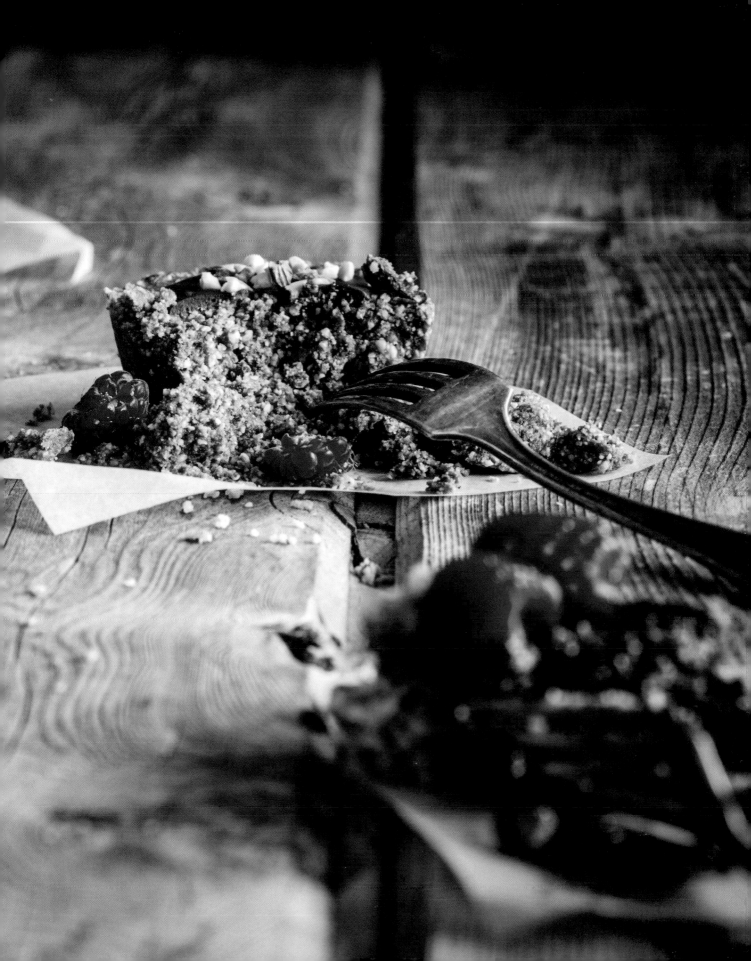

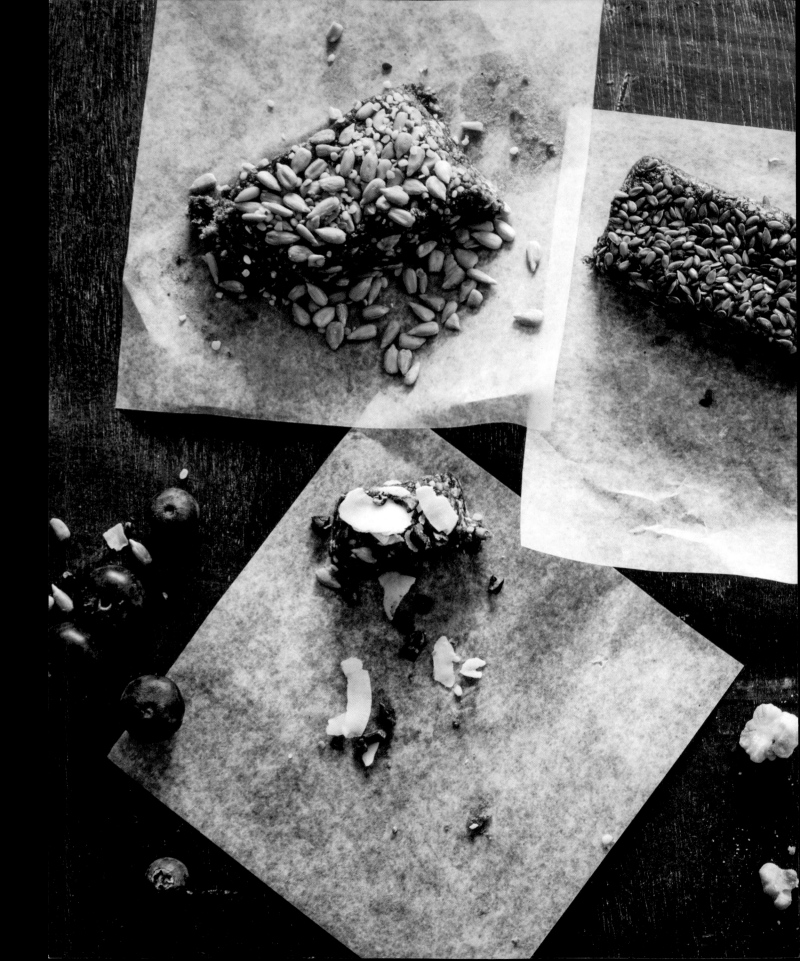

THRIVE SPORT RECIPES

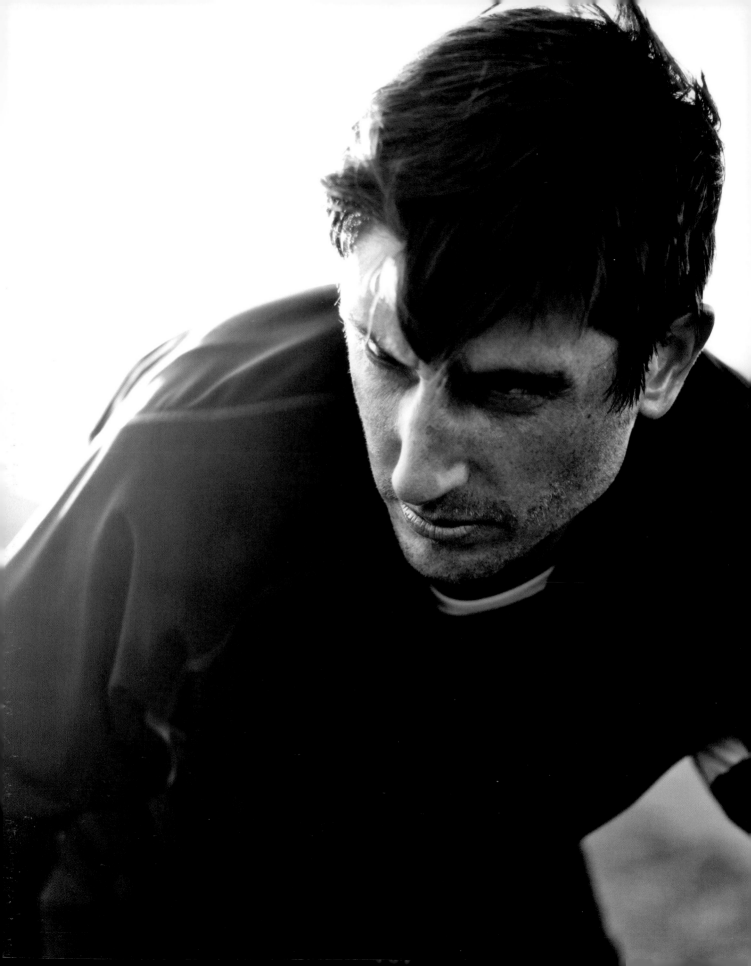

High-net-gain nutrition is one of the key elements of living a life of sustained energy. And as an athlete, the benefits of high-net-gain nutrition become even greater. In this section, I've compiled a few of my favorite sport-specific recipes, to be eaten a short time before a workout, during, or immediately after.

Being well fueled before and during training will of course allow for a better-quality workout, which translates into gains being realized in less time. But the challenge then becomes how to get adequate fuel into your system while spending the least amount of digestive energy. After all, when the digestive system has to kick in and work harder to process food, less blood is available to circulate throughout the arms and legs, which means a reduced amount of oxygen being delivered to the extremities and less metabolic waste product being removed. This situation is obviously not desirable. And so I created these recipes, which can be digested with ease yet still meet the fueling requirements of the high-achieving athlete.

When I first began racing Ironman triathlons seriously, I was meticulous about fully testing my planned race-day fuel strategy during rigorous training sessions—dry runs, so to speak. But although the tests often indicated that I was on track, race day frequently turned out to be a whole different scenario. I simply wasn't able to digest the food; it just sat in my stomach. I was puzzled. How was it that my digestive system worked during training, and even in mock race settings, yet essentially shut down in a real race?

Adrenaline. As I learned, when the excitement of race day kicks in—combined with butterflies—the result is a system flooded with the hormone adrenaline. That's not necessarily a bad thing. Adrenaline sharpens your focus and enhances your physical ability to perform. However, it also wreaks havoc on the digestive system—as I'd discovered. With this newfound knowledge, I was able to formulate recipes with enhanced digestive ease in mind. We now offer many of them at Thrive Energy Lab.

As with pre-workout fuel, post-workout nutrition also ought to be easy to digest. Immediately after a workout, having to digest food that requires an inordinate amount of energy to be spent will reduce the amount of energy that can be allocated toward recovery. That's one of the reasons I suggest drinking a smoothie immediately after a workout (such as the one on page 273), but I've also included an easily digestible high-net-gain cereal as an alternative (page 269).

I've divided these sport-specific recipes into three categories: Prepare, Sustain, and Recover.

"Optimized nutrition,
optimized performance."

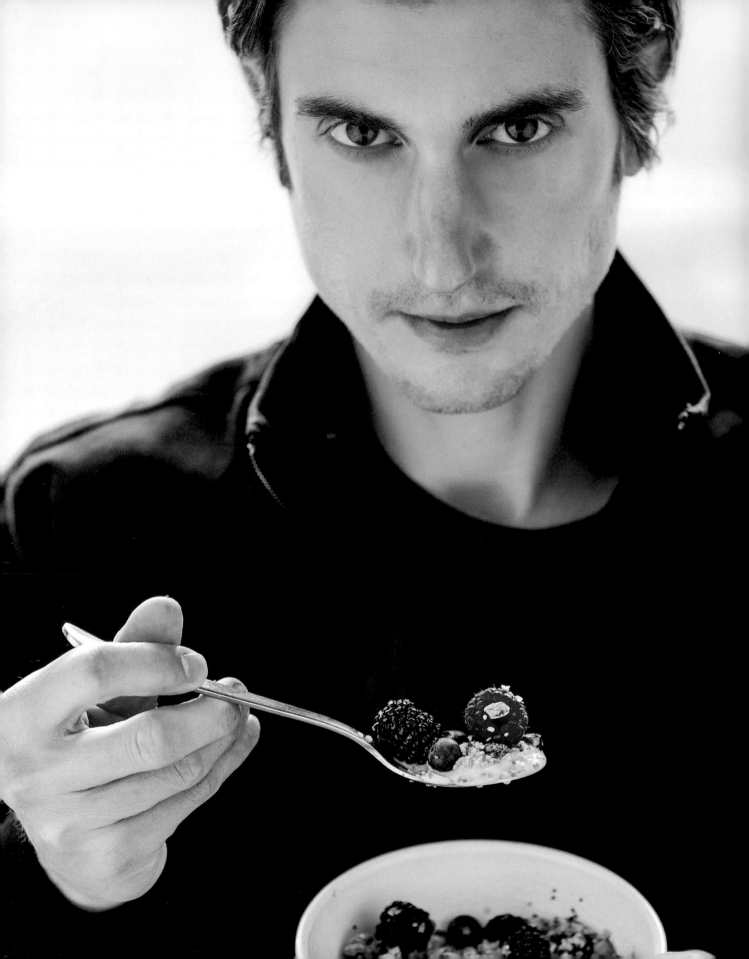

BLUEBERRY CACAO PRE-WORKOUT PERFORMANCE CEREAL

This cereal is an ideal sustaining fuel for workouts that will exceed 90 minutes. The natural serotonin release from the cacao will help you stay mentally focused. The macronutrients are synergistically combined to deliver a steady release of energy for sustained performance. The dates provide immediate energy, and then the coconut nectar will kick in just as the glucose wears off—no energy dip will occur. The oats will prolong your muscles' ability to function efficiently. And, if you're performing a lower intensity, longer workout, the flax and chia will enhance your body's ability to burn fat as fuel. If you want to turbocharge your cereal, add green tea or matcha powder. Serves 5/Makes 4 cups (1 L)

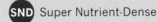 **GF** Gluten-Free   **PR** Protein-Rich   **SND** Super Nutrient-Dense

Prep Time: 8 minutes

1 cup (250 mL) gluten-free rolled oats

½ cup (125 mL) fresh or frozen blueberries

3 large Medjool dates, pitted and chopped

½ cup (125 mL) chopped raw almonds

½ cup (125 mL) sunflower seeds

½ cup (125 mL) ground flaxseed

½ cup (125 mL) chia seeds

½ cup (125 mL) unhulled sesame seeds

2 tbsp (30 mL) cacao nibs

¼ tsp (1 mL) sea salt

¼ cup (60 mL) virgin coconut oil, melted

¼ cup (60 mL) coconut nectar

2 tbsp (30 mL) water

2 tbsp (30 mL) matcha green tea powder (turbocharge option)

4 tsp (20 mL) cayenne pepper (optional)

Preheat oven to 250°F (120°C).

In a large bowl, combine the oats, blueberries, dates, almonds, sunflower seeds, flaxseed, chia seeds, sesame seeds, cacao nibs, and sea salt. Stir until well combined. In a small bowl, stir together the coconut oil, coconut nectar, water, green tea powder (if using), and cayenne (if using).

Add the wet ingredients to the dry ingredients. Mix well. Spread evenly on a baking sheet.

Bake, stirring once halfway through, for 50 to 65 minutes, depending on how much crunch you like. Let cool on the baking sheet. Break up before storing.

· ·

- Top with easily digestible, antioxidant-rich berries such as blackberries and raspberries.
- The optional cayenne increases blood flow and therefore speeds the uptake of nutrients.
- Keeps in an open container, refrigerated, for up to 2 weeks.

ACAI BERRY PRE-WORKOUT ENERGIZER

Designed to be consumed about 40 minutes before a longer or especially intense workout, this easy-to-digest pre-workout fuel will provide your muscles with clean-burning carbs to carry you through the toughest of workouts. Since it's in liquid form it will digest easily and therefore reduces the risk of a dreaded side stitch. Also, pineapple is high in a digestive enzyme called bromelain that further assists with digestibility. In addition, the Vega Sport Pre-Workout Energizer will give your fat metabolism a boost with its green tea and yerba mate, enabling your body to burn more body fat while sparing muscle glycogen, thereby directly boosting endurance. Serves 1/Makes 2¼ cups (550 mL)

GF Gluten-Free   **SND** Super Nutrient-Dense

Prep Time: 2 to 3 minutes • **Special Equipment:** high-speed blender

In a blender, combine all the ingredients except the ice. Add ice to about 1 inch (2.5 cm) above the liquid line. Blend on high speed until smooth.

....

- If using frozen fruit, use less ice.
- The agave is recommended if you're planning a workout that will exceed 3 hours.

4 fresh or frozen strawberries

⅓ cup (75 mL) chopped pineapple

¼ cup (60 mL) fresh or frozen blueberries

1 scoop acai berry–flavor Vega Sport Pre-Workout Energizer

½ cup (125 mL) coconut water

½ cup (125 mL) acai berry juice

1 tbsp (15 mL) agave nectar or maple syrup (optional)

About 2 cups (500 mL) ice cubes

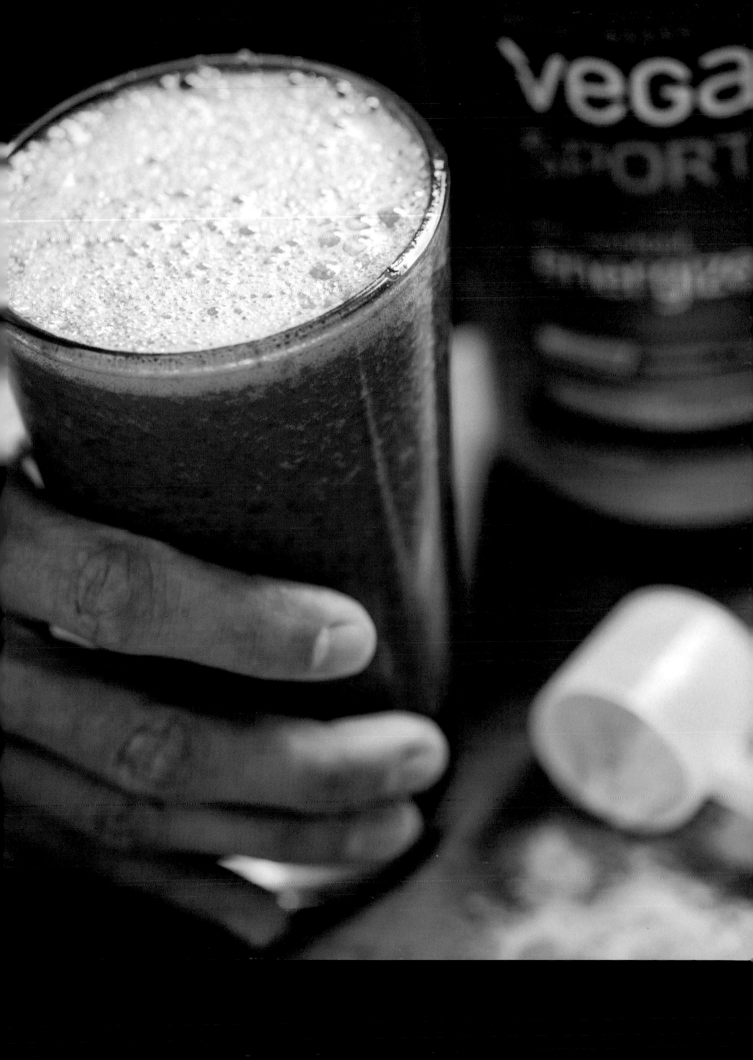

BLUEBERRY BUCKWHEAT ENERGY BARS

These bars are ideal for sustaining physical activity. I have synergistically combined ingredients that will provide immediate and sustained energy, while being easy to digest.

I include a small amount of palm sugar, not to make the bars sweeter, but rather as a functional fuel. Palm sugar has a low glycemic index, meaning it will enter the bloodstream gradually, providing sustained energy. This, combined with the dates, which are primarily glucose and provide immediate energy, results in a functional, sustainable energy bar. **Makes about 1 dozen bars**

R Raw   **GF** Gluten-Free   **PR** Protein-Rich

Prep Time: 5 minutes • **Special Equipment:** food processor

1 cup (250 mL) pitted and soaked Medjool dates

¼ cup (60 mL) fresh or frozen blueberries

¼ cup (60 mL) whole raw walnuts

¼ cup (60 mL) ground flaxseed

¼ cup (60 mL) unhulled hemp seeds

¼ cup (60 mL) hemp protein or berry-flavor Vega Sport Performance Protein

1 tbsp (15 mL) coconut palm sugar

Sea salt

½ cup (125 mL) sprouted or cooked buckwheat (optional)

¼ cup (60 mL) chopped walnuts

½ cup (125 mL) frozen blueberries

In a food processer, combine the dates, ¼ cup (60 mL) fresh or frozen blueberries, whole walnuts, flaxseed, hemp seeds, hemp protein, palm sugar, and salt to taste. Process until desired texture is reached. The less you process, the crunchier the bar will be.

Transfer mixture to a bowl and knead in the buckwheat (if using), chopped walnuts, and blueberries with your hands (or pulse a couple of times to get a coarse blend).

To shape into balls: use a spoon or your hands to scoop the mixture (however much you like to make 1 ball) and roll between your palms.

To shape into bars: turn mixture out onto a work surface. Flatten with your hands. Place a sheet of plastic wrap on top, then roll with a rolling pin to desired thickness. Cut into bars.

Alternatively, form the mixture into a brick, then cut into slices. Or press the mixture into a baking dish lined with parchment paper, refrigerate for about 5 hours, and slice into bars. As the bars dry in the fridge, they become easier to handle and slice.

....

- **Keep in a sealed container, refrigerated, or individually wrap in plastic wrap and freeze. Because of the fatty acids, the bars will not freeze solid and can therefore be eaten straight from the freezer.**
- **For variation, use ¾ cup (175 mL) of sprouted whole flax seeds, coconut shavings, or sunflower seeds as toppings when you form the bars.**

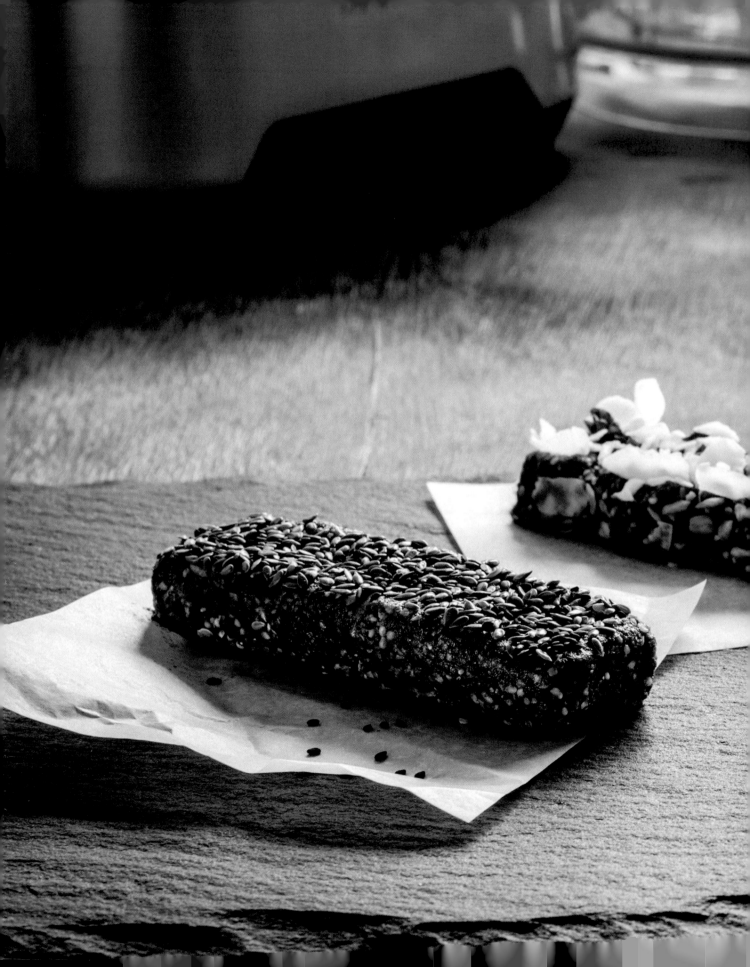

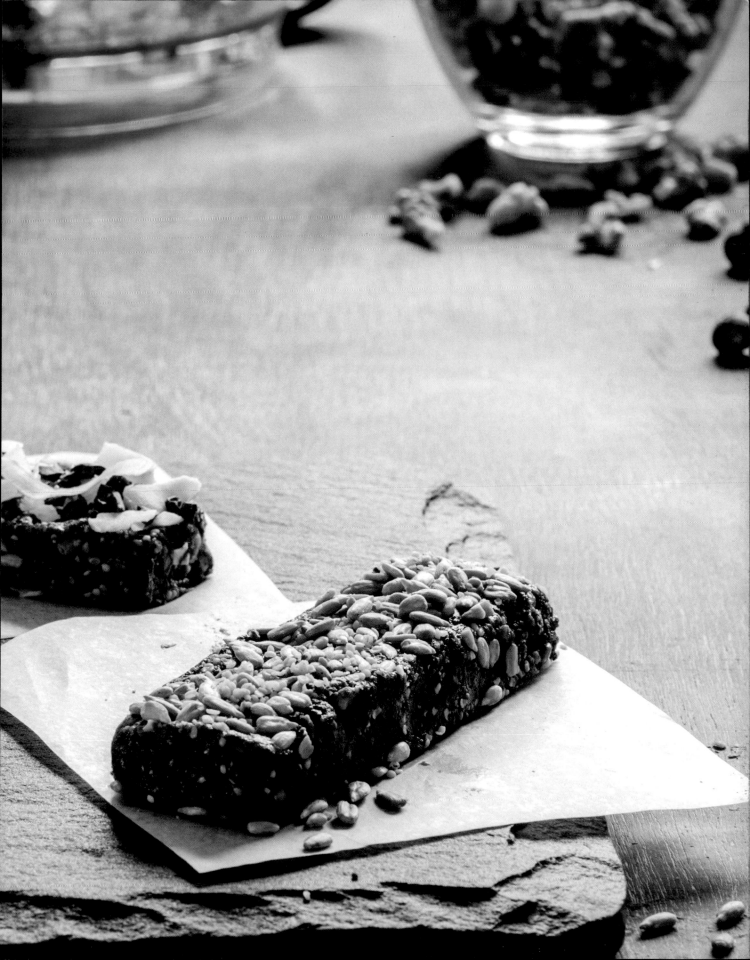

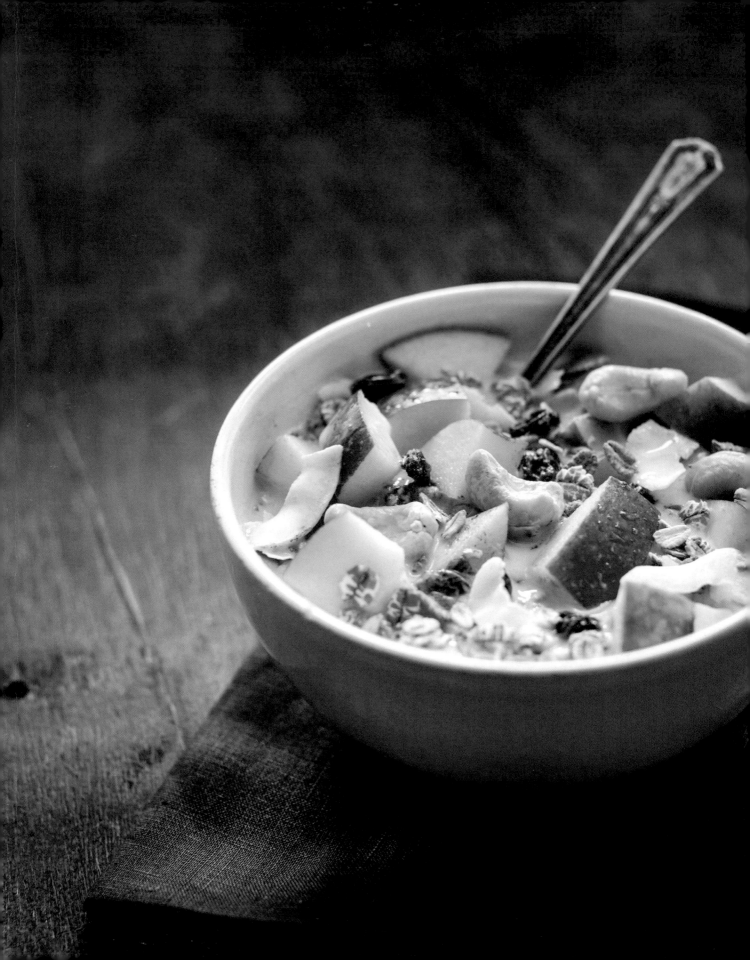

COCONUT MANGO RECOVERY CEREAL

Carbohydrate from the mango, oats, dates, and coconut nectar will restock depleted glycogen stores; the essential fatty acids from the flax, cashews, and chia will enhance fat metabolism; and the high-quality, alkaline-forming protein from the nuts, seeds, almond milk, and optional Vega Sport Performance Protein powder will reduce inflammation and instigate protein synthesis. Serves 5/Makes 4 cups (1 L)

GF Gluten-Free   **PR** Protein-Rich

Prep Time: 5 minutes

Preheat oven to 250°F (120°C).

In a medium bowl, combine the mango, dates, oats, cashews, flaxseed, chia seeds, sesame seeds, sunflower seeds, shredded coconut, cacao nibs, and sea salt. Stir until well combined.

In a small bowl, stir together the coconut oil, coconut nectar, and water.

Add the wet ingredients to the dry ingredients. Mix well. Spread evenly on a baking sheet.

Bake, stirring once halfway through, for 50 to 65 minutes, depending on how much crunch you like. Let cool on the baking sheet. Break up before storing.

....

- Add finely grated fresh ginger on top to reduce inflammation.
- Top with diced apples that are rich in pectin and will assist mineral (electrolyte) absorption. This is important post-workout to regain full hydration.
- This cereal can be served with almond milk (page 23) or Vega Sport Performance Protein.
- Keeps in an open container, refrigerated, for up to 2 weeks.

½ large mango, peeled and diced

3 large Medjool dates, pitted and diced

1 cup (250 mL) gluten-free rolled oats

½ cup (125 mL) raw cashews

½ cup (125 mL) ground flaxseed

½ cup (125 mL) chia seeds

½ cup (125 mL) unhulled sesame seeds

½ cup (125 mL) sunflower seeds

2 tbsp (30 mL) unsweetened shredded coconut

2 tbsp (30 mL) cacao nibs

¼ tsp (1 mL) sea salt

¼ cup (60 mL) virgin coconut oil, melted

¼ cup (60 mL) coconut nectar

2 tbsp (30 mL) water

COOKIES & CREAM RECOVERY SMOOTHIE

Ideal for strength athletes in pursuit of building lean mass, this recovery smoothie is a delicious way to feed your fatigued muscles while reducing inflammation and oxidative damage to your cells. Popularized at the Thrive Energy Lab by those who just spent themselves at the gym. Serves 1/Makes 2¼ cups (550 mL)

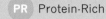 **GF** Gluten-Free   **SND** Super Nutrient-Dense   **PR** Protein-Rich

---

Prep Time: 2 minutes • **Special Equipment:** high-speed blender

In a blender, combine all the ingredients except the ice. Add ice to about 1 inch (2.5 cm) above the liquid line. Blend on high speed until smooth and creamy.

• **The optional agave is suggested if your workout has exceeded 90 minutes.**

2 tbsp (30 mL) raw cashews

2 tbsp (30 mL) vegan dark chocolate chips

1 tbsp (15 mL) cacao nibs

1 tbsp (15 mL) raw cashew butter

1 tbsp (15 mL) pitted and chopped Medjool dates

1 scoop vanilla Vega Sport Performance Protein

1 cup (250 mL) unsweetened almond milk (or homemade, page 23)

¼ cup (60 mL) agave nectar or maple syrup (optional)

About 2 cups (500 mL) ice cubes

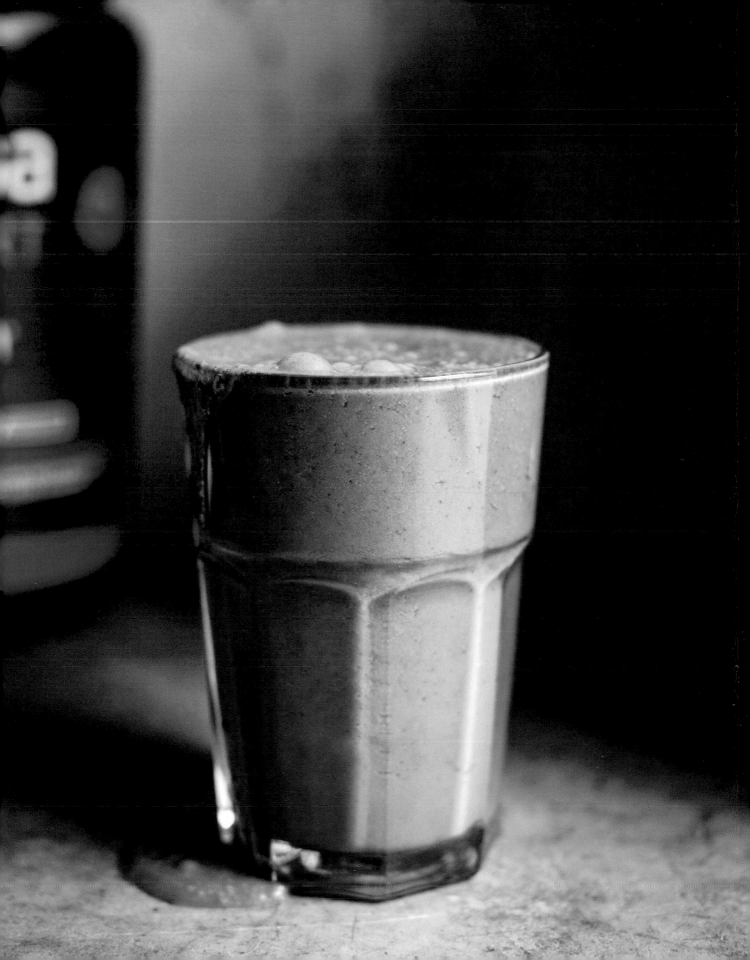

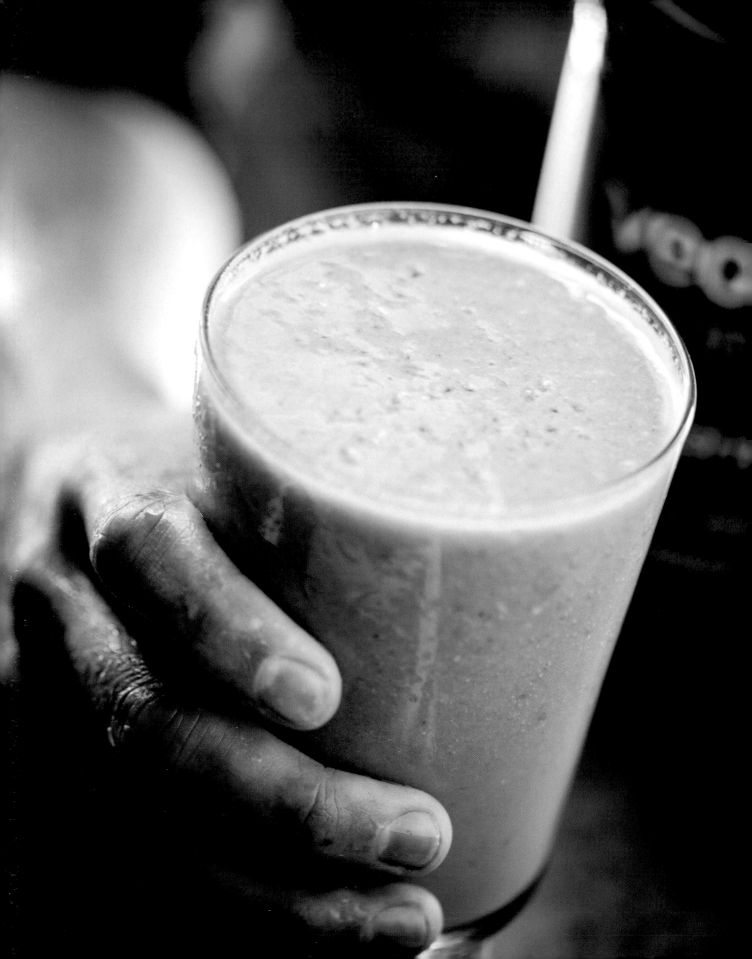

GOJI APPLE-BERRY RECOVERY SMOOTHIE

Designed to be consumed immediately after either a long or an intense workout, this recovery drink will help speed glycogen replenishment, reduce oxidization of the cells, reduce inflammation, lower cortisol, restore electrolyte balance, boost immune function, and instigate protein synthesis. And because of this, your next workout will be of higher quality, leading you to improve at a faster rate as an athlete. At the Thrive Energy Lab, this is a favorite of cyclists who visit on their way home from a long Sunday ride. Serves 1/Makes 1¾ cups (425 mL)

 Gluten-Free    Super Nutrient-Dense

---

Prep Time: 2 to 3 minutes • **Special Equipment:** high-speed blender

In a blender, combine all the ingredients except the ice. Add ice to about 1 inch (2.5 cm) above the liquid line. Blend on high speed until smooth and creamy.

....

• If using frozen fruit, use less ice.

¼ cup (60 mL) blueberries

¼ cup (60 mL) raspberries

1 scoop Vega apple-berry recovery powder

½ cup (125 mL) acai berry juice

½ cup (125 mL) coconut water

1 Medjool date

3 tbsp (45 mL) fresh orange juice

1 tsp (5 mL) goji berries

2 cups (500 mL) ice

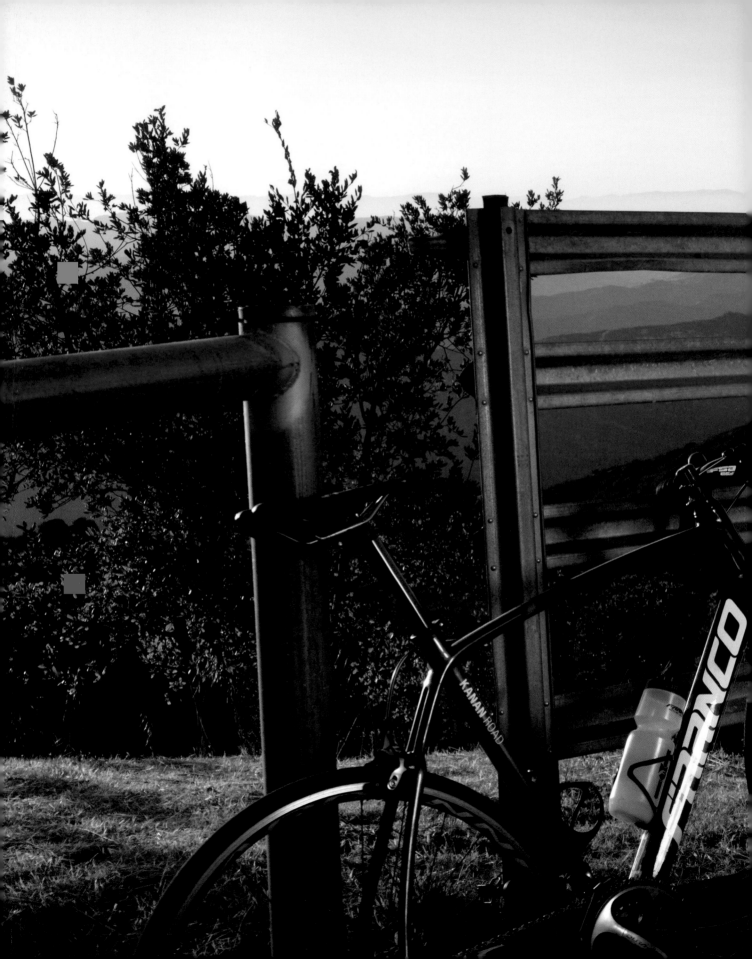

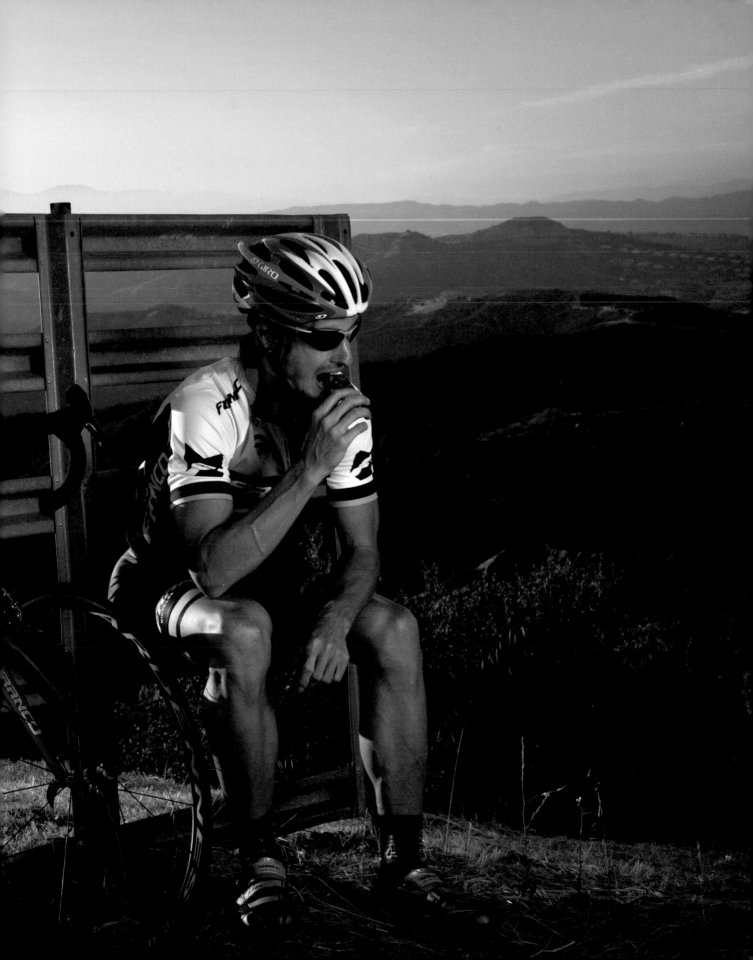

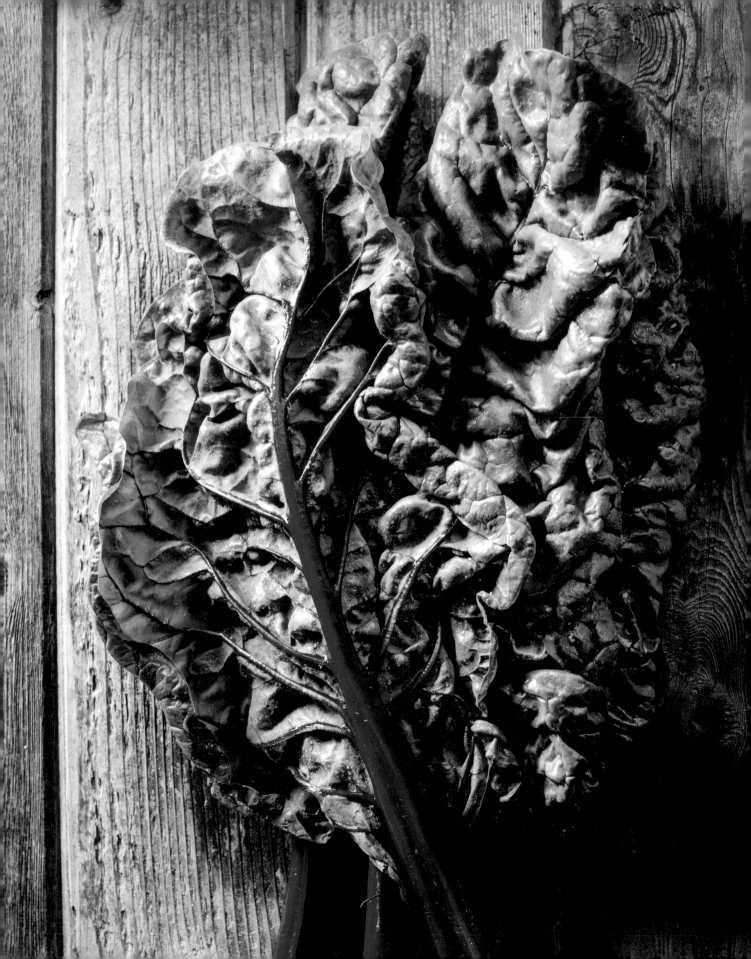

TRANSITIONAL MEAL PLAN

Breakfast: Cashew Berry French Toast (page 49)

Snack: Chocolate Chip French Vanilla Smoothie (page 189)

Lunch: Reuben Sandwich (page 84)

Snack: Pecan Bars (page 231)

Dinner: Avocado, Black Bean & Chipotle Burger with Roasted Red Pepper & Sweet Potato Soup (pages 98 and 117)

Dessert: Chocolate Cacao Cupcakes (page 234)

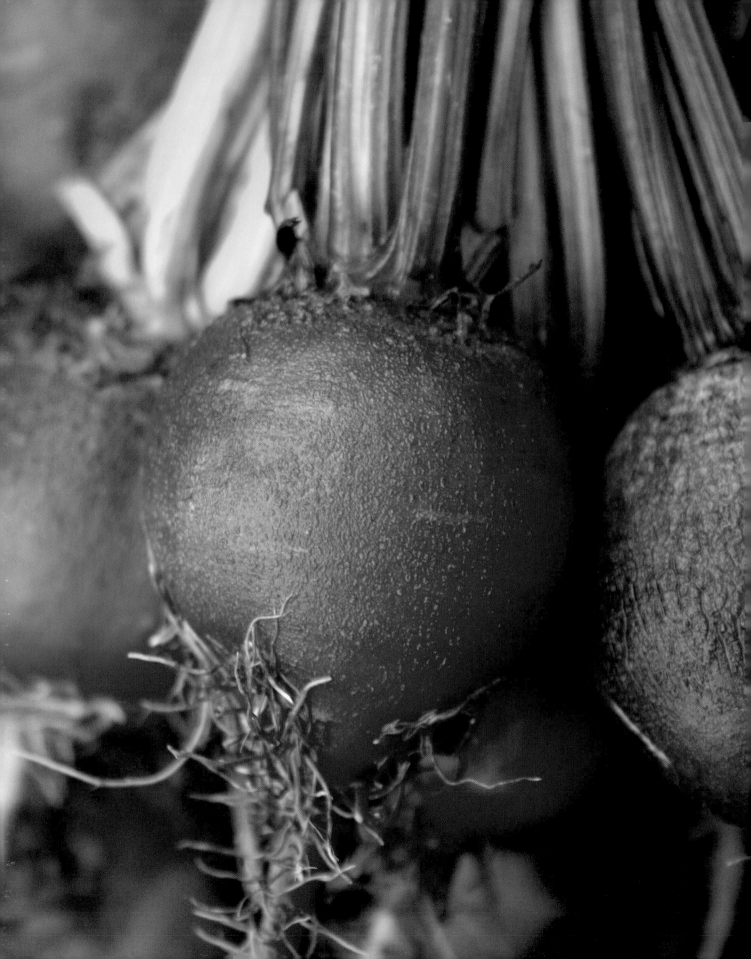

STANDARD MEAL PLAN

Pre-workout: Acai Berry Pre-Workout Energizer (page 262)
**(for 30 to 60 minutes of light to moderate training—if longer
duration or more intense, see Athletic Meal Plan example)**

Post-workout: Cookies & Cream Recovery Smoothie (page 270) *or*
Coconut Mango Recovery Cereal (page 269)

Lunch: Quinoa Tabbouleh Salad (page 143)

Snack: Kale Mojito (page 171)

**Dinner: Pad Thai Rice Noodle Bowl
with raw kelp noodle option** (page 158)

Snack: apple and raw walnuts

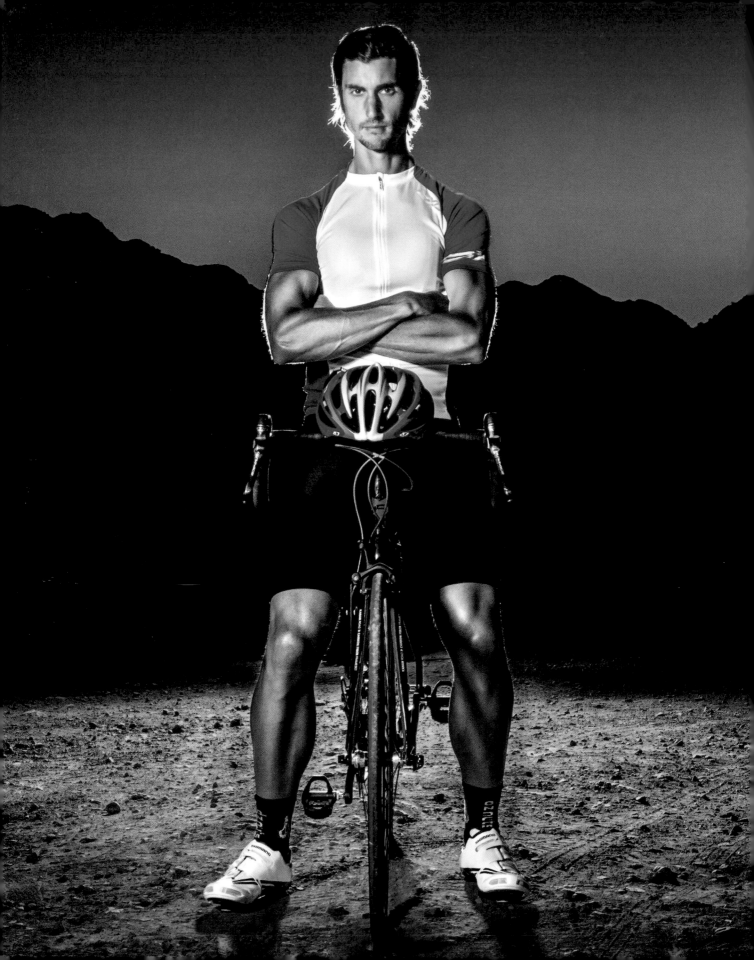

ATHLETIC MEAL PLAN

Pre-workout: **Acai Berry Pre-Workout Energizer** (page 262) *or*
Blueberry Cacao Pre-Workout Performance Cereal (page 261)
(workout longer than 60 minutes or of above average intensity)

Post-workout: **Goji Apple-Berry Recovery Smoothie** (page 273)

Snack: Chocolate-Almond Decadence (page 175)

Lunch: A.L.T. Avocado, Lettuce & Tomato Sandwich (page 83)

Snack: fresh fruit and raw nuts or seeds

Dinner: Avocado & Kelp Noodle Salad (page 133)

Dessert: Raspberry Chocolate Pomegranate Tart (page 240)

Snack: Kale Chips (page 59)

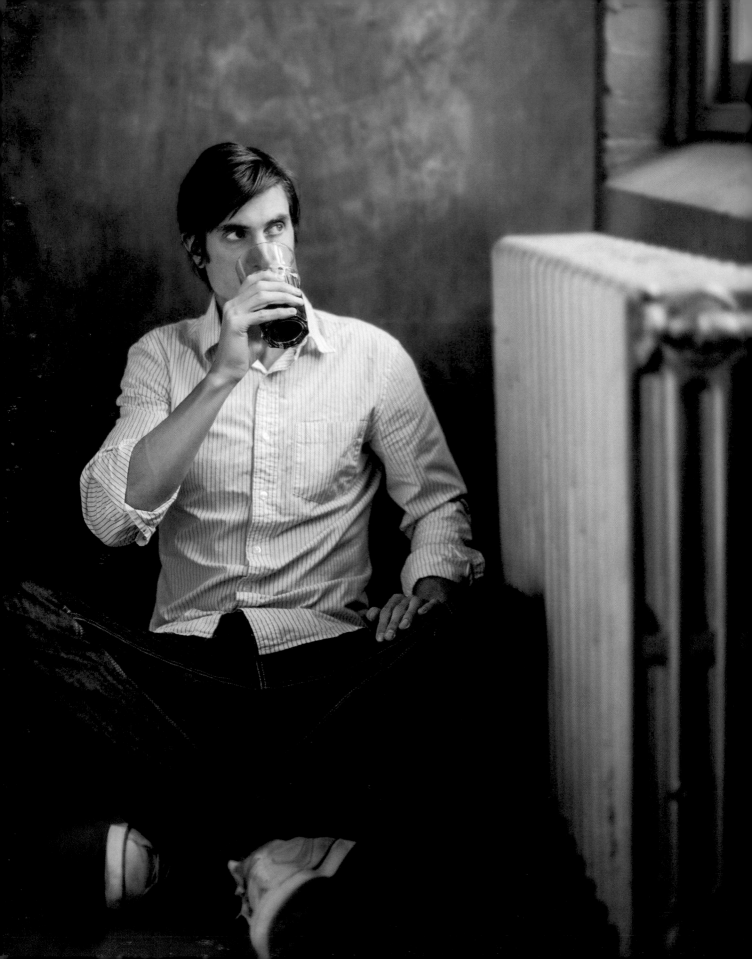

Thanks

Charles Chang—If I know how to do it and it has something to do with anything other than swimming, cycling, running, eating, or sleeping, I learned it from Charles. We met in my seventh year of professional Ironman racing, which I had done full-time since high school. So my skill set was limited, to say the least. But I had come up with a functional nutritional shake that I developed over the years to help speed recovery between workouts. And Charles—having started a natural nutrition company just a few years prior—took an interest. We became friends, and after only a few conversations, Charles suggested I write a book—about my plant-based performance nutrition philosophy that had worked well for me—and travel around speaking about it. Never having written a word, nor spoken to an audience, I took his suggestion as a vote of confidence. Clearly Charles believed in the value of my message and saw potential in me as a vessel to communicate it. This led me to writing my first book that would develop into the Thrive book series. We then partnered and created the Vega line of nutritional products.

Andrea Magyar—For her foresight and believing that writing a "vegan book for non-vegans" actually made sense. Thank you for taking a chance on the series and being a true pleasure to work with every step of the way.

Robert Mackwood—For helping me navigate the publishing world from the very beginning.

Jonnie Karan and his staff at Thrive Energy Lab in Waterloo, Ontario, for making these recipes possible

Jonnie Karan—Founder and creator of the Thrive Energy Lab recipes
Stephanie Spencer—Created and tested drink recipes
Rhianne Byron—Created and tested dessert recipes
Vanessa Lekun—Created and tested food recipes

Products We Use at Thrive Energy Lab

Vega

Over the past 10 years, the Vega line of nutritional products has grown considerably. Born in 2004 from an always-improving formula I've been making for myself since I was a teenager, Vega One is an all-in-one nutritional shake I created to help speed recovery after training. The Vega line now includes bars, as well as a separate Vega Sport line that I formulated specifically for athletes and anyone aspiring to boost athletic performance. Vega products are plant-based, free of common allergens (no wheat, yeast, gluten, corn, soy, or dairy), and natural. So, as you would expect, we use the Vega line exclusively at Thrive Energy Lab.
myvega.com
vegasport.com

Silver Hills Bakery

I've been eating Silver Hills sprouted bread since the early 1990s. When I first made the switch to plant-based eating in 1990, my mum was concerned that I wouldn't get enough protein, so she bought me a loaf of Silver Hills Squirrely bread. I've had it as a staple in my diet every since. Silver Hills is unique in that their bread is not made of flour, but rather sprouted whole grains. Many don't realize it, but sprouted grain offers quite a large amount of complete protein. One slice of Silver Hills bread has 6 to 7 grams of protein (a medium sized egg has 6 grams), so it's an easy way to add protein to your diet. That's why we use it exclusively at Thrive Energy Lab. Silver Hills also makes several rice-based gluten-free options as well.
silverhillsbakery.ca

Breville

Breville makes exceptionally durable, well-designed, functional appliances. Even their consumer models are of commercial strength and quality. That's why we exclusively use their whole range of appliances at Thrive Energy Lab. Juicers, blenders, food processors, grills, and toaster ovens, Breville makes them all. We highly recommended them.
brevilleusa.com

Index

C